Setting Boundaries® with Your Adult Children

This book will launch a brand new beginning in your life. You may feel you are in a desert place right now as you struggle with a parenting crisis, but be alert! There's a stream in the wasteland—and you can begin making hope-filled choices that will forever change your future for the better.

—**Carol Kent,**
speaker and author of *When I Lay My Isaac Down*
and *A New Kind of Normal*

No one knows better the pain of dealing with adult children who have lost their way better than the parents of those without boundaries. Sometimes it feels as though the setting of these boundaries is more difficult than living with the anxiety, stress, and heartache, but that's not so. Allison Bottke, writing through her own hurt and experience, has compiled a masterpiece of advice. She doesn't just tell you or show you how it's done. She walks along beside you.

—**Eva Marie Everson & Jessica Everson,**
authors of *Sex, Lies, and the Media*
and *Sex, Lies, and High School*

Lack of boundaries with adult children is a worldwide epidemic with catastrophic consequences. Allison shares not only her experience as a parent who has traveled this painful road, but gives readers concrete tools to stop the insanity and start living a life of hope and healing. *Setting Boundaries with Your Adult Children* is destined to be the official resource of hope for countless parents and grandparents.

—**Heather Gemmen Wilson,**
author of *Startling Beauty: My Journey
from Rape to Restoration*

Allison Bottke has stepped forward in a courageous, straight-from-the-heart manner and dealt with an issue that has plagued parents since the dawn of time: setting (and enforcing) boundaries for rebellious adult children. Having been not only a parent but a pastor who faced this issue countless times, I am excited to see that a mother who has wrestled with demons to see her child delivered has written a heartfelt yet practical book of advice and encouragement that will bless each and every one who reads it.

—**Kathi Macias,**
author of 20 books, including *Mothers of the Bible
Speak to Mothers Today*

Setting Boundaries with Your Adult Children is an incredible resource, an absolutely must-have book for parents with adult children. It will help you so much to understand where your adult children are in their own journey and how to transition in a healthy way in setting new boundaries. This book will inspire you, encourage you, and prepare you to handle this season in the parenting process.

—Pastor Chuck Angel,
Harvest Church, Fort Worth, TX

To some readers this book will arrive just in time, releasing them from the bondage of a present crisis. To others, this book will serve as a how-to manual when the unwanted crisis comes knocking. To many, this timely teaching will serve as a mirror, exposing lies and revealing the truth. But Allison Bottke doesn't leave us sulking at our reflection. In *Setting Boundaries with Your Adult Children*, she places within our hands a prescription. When filled and faithfully followed, her writing will bring hope and healing.

—Pastor Steve Hill,
Heartland World Ministries Church,
Las Colinas, TX

I have talked with many parents who know they need boundaries with both their adult and adolescent kids. They are apprehensive about setting limits and fearful of enforcing them. Readers will identify with Allison. She offers many helpful suggestions on establishing and implementing workable boundaries that will bring harmony back to families. I recommend her book to all parents.

—Pastor Larry Bodmer,
Director of Biblical Counseling,
Overlake Christian Church, Redmond, WA

Setting Boundaries® with Difficult People

In her typical insightful fashion, Allison Bottke has given us a valuable and practical guide for *Setting Boundaries with Difficult People*. Well organized, powerfully written, thoughtful, challenging, and helpful for everyday living, this excellent volume is a keeper—a reference you'll refer to repeatedly as you encounter those inevitable aggravating relationships. Get it. Read it. Use it! And celebrate your less-stressful life.

—Mary Hollingsworth,
Bestselling Author and Managing Director,
Creative Enterprises Studio

Once again Allison Bottke has written an amazing masterpiece. *Setting Boundaries with Difficult People* is a challenge in life that everyone has to deal with. It is obvious this book was bathed in fervent prayer. Once you begin to read this book, you will not want to put it down.

—**Sharon Hill,**
Founder, OnCall Prayer.org
and author of the *OnCall Prayer Journal*

Setting Boundaries with Difficult People touches the heart of the matter in this inspired expression of help and hope for all who face challenging relationships in life. The author's ability to weave together the story, the resources, and the Christian worldview is brilliant!

—**Suellen Roberts,**
Founder & President,
Christian Women in Media Association

Unless you live in complete isolation as a hermit (and who does?), you have some difficult people in your life (family, coworkers, professional colleagues, friends, you name it). In easy-to-understand, straightforward teaching, Allison Bottke gives readers critical relationship tools in *Setting Boundaries with Difficult People,* providing excellent insight and step-by-step action for every reader. I highly recommend this book. In fact, you should probably buy at least two of them—one for yourself and one to give to someone else. It is that good.

—**Terry Whalin,**
editor and writer

Allison Bottke has written a helpful and inspiring book on how to live with and manage difficult relationships at home, at work, in our community. We all have people in our lives who challenge us, and yet God loves them as much as He loves us! So the task is to be kind, loving, grace filled and firm about how we wish to be treated. After reading this book you'll be well-equipped to do all of these things.

—**Karen O'Connor,**
author of *Help, Lord! I'm Having a Senior Moment*

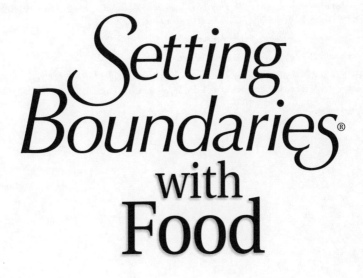

Setting *Boundaries*® with Food

ALLISON BOTTKE

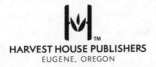

HARVEST HOUSE PUBLISHERS
EUGENE, OREGON

SETTING BOUNDARIES® WITH FOOD
Copyright © 2012 by Allison Bottke
Published by Harvest House Publishers
Eugene, Oregon 97402
www.harvesthousepublishers.com

Library of Congress Cataloging-in-Publication Data
    Bottke, Allison.
    Setting boundaries with food / Allison Bottke.
        p. cm.
    Includes bibliographical references
    ISBN 978-0-7369-2694-2 (pbk.)
    ISBN 978-0-7369-4290-4 (eBook)
    1. Food—Religious aspects—Christianity. I. Title.
    BR115.N87B68 2012
    241'.68—dc23
                                                                2011051600

For Pastor Victor Constien

Thank you for being salt and light in the lives of so many, and for illuminating my path so that I might come to know the Lord as my God.

When I dedicated my life to a heavenly Father who would protect, guide, and love me unconditionally, you felt called to present Psalm 27:1 as a guiding scripture for my life.

Only God in His infinite wisdom, grace, and mercy could have known the power this Word would have on my life.

"The Lord is my light and my salvation—whom shall I fear? The Lord is the stronghold of my life— of whom shall I be afraid?" (NIV)

May God continue to richly bless your life as you have blessed mine.

A mighty fortress is our God!

Contents

Foreword
by Dr. Chuck and Jill Angel
Harvest Church, Fort Worth, Texas

Four feet eight and a half inches. That's the standard width of train tracks in the United States. Regardless if a train is traveling from Miami to New York, or Ft. Worth to Chicago, it's rolling down a set of rails that are spaced at the same distance mile after mile. To reach its destination, it really doesn't matter what logo happens to be on the side of the train or if the cargo is holiday bound passengers or West Virginia coal. Rather it's all about four feet eight and a half inches of reliably spaced rails.

A life message is a heart cry that God gives to a person who has come to know a hard-learned lesson plumbed out of the depths of their own life experience...and candidly often-painful experience. What is gained from that pain and shared with others becomes a living word. It hits the soul with such comfort. It makes sense in our mind. It always sounds fresh. It's always on time. And, for author Allison Bottke, she has found her life message. It's all about setting healthy boundaries, giving people dependable, reliable rails to run on. It's her four feet eight and a half inches of life-changing truth!

In her latest book, Allison applies boundaries to the subject of food. When she handed me the manuscript I honestly thought: "I don't want to read this." I mean I love and need boundaries when it comes to people but I really don't want anything to keep me from something that's the source of so much comfort and pleasure. Why would anyone in their right mind want a border that keeps them at a distance from a chilled Girl Scout Thin Mint?

You are probably a lot like me. As a pastor I live with a fair amount of pressure. I'm familiar with coping with a wide range of high expectations. The more pressure I feel the more subconsciously I drift toward the fridge. It feels very natural. In fact it's even how I have rewarded my children. When a good grade is achieved we go get ice cream. When their behavior was pleasant, I'd reward them with a special treat. Where did that come from? Why was food as a reward so engrained? But more importantly how could I stop?

Chapter seven was pure revelation for me. God is love—not food! Truth so simple and profound helped me to see and understand how I had made a deep long-standing connection with food. I knew that Jesus had promised to offer something to the soul that could quench its thirst. In fact He said "you will never become thirsty again" (John 4:14). Now I know Jesus, but I found myself continuously hungry, so what was I not getting? Allison helped me get to the heart of the matter!

No matter why you picked up this book, you are going to find that her candid story, her devotion to truth, and her compassionate counsel will help you. This is a wonderful woman with a life message we need to hear. Her heart cry will inspire you, comfort you, and call you to new levels of freedom and joy!

Dr. Chuck Angel, Senior Pastor,
Harvest Church, Fort Worth, Texas

I love the analogy my husband has written about train tracks and Allison's passion to provide reliable rails in the form of healthy boundaries to help us navigate difficult relationships in our lives. From *Setting Boundaries with Your Adult Children* to *Setting Boundaries with Difficult People*, it's clear that God has placed a powerful call on Allison's heart.

In *Setting Boundaries with Food*, I also love the refreshing and no-holds-barred way Allison brings to light a topic that doesn't get much dialog in the church—gluttony.

Since we don't want to hurt feelings or cause people to feel worse, sometimes we avoid certain topics and this is one that is glazed over quite often. I love her healthy approach to what God says about this very serious issue that plagues many of us.

Being the mother of three daughters and one son I am quite familiar with the delicacy of talking about overeating. It seems like I have no problem teaching our children other biblical principles like: Don't lie, don't steal, and don't gossip. But when it comes to "don't overeat or use food as comfort" I have always struggled for fear they would resent me, which would lead to more eating and result in unhealthy weight gain. As a teenager I struggled with my weight and know how it feels to be called fat and I don't want that for my daughters or my son.

After reading Allison's relevant, timely, and tell-it-like-it-is book on boundaries with food, I have gained a newfound urgency to teach my kids that food is not love, God is, and to find their ultimate acceptance in Christ. In one of his sermon messages last year I agreed when Chuck said that *Setting Boundaries with Your Adult Children* was a must-read for every parent and grandparent. I'm going to add *Setting Boundaries with Food* to that must-read list, and it will be on the required reading list for my children, without a doubt! It would have saved me a lot of pain if I had read this as a young girl.

I thank God for Allison's authentic and transparent openness with her story. It is powerful and has the potential to change and save thousands from a life of bondage to food.

Jill Angel, Wife and Executive Assistant to Pastor Chuck
Harvest Church, Fort Worth, Texas

Introduction

For many years my life was a never-ending drama of crisis after crisis revolving around my drug-addicted son. It was absolute insanity—and it was not how God intended for me (or any parent) to live.

Before I was able to eventually write *Setting Boundaries with Your Adult Children*, the first book in the Setting Boundaries® series, I had to first recognize my own enabling patterns of behavior and put a stop to the part I had played in repeatedly accepting the vicious cycle of irresponsible behavior in my son's life. Before God could use me to help others find sanity, I first had to learn how to stop trying to fix the mess my son was making of his life and fix the mess I had made of my own.

As I developed what I call the Six Steps to SANITY in dealing with my son, I began to realize the futility of harboring negative feelings of guilt, frustration, anger, fear, and inadequacy. Those destructive emotions only hindered my ability to resolve the daily drama of those years. Instead, I began to focus on developing new strengths that helped me break free from the bondage of the poor choices my son was making. I learned I had to make better choices myself.

Today, thousands of parents and grandparents around the world have joined me in finding freedom from the exhausting cycle of enabling our adult children. Together we have found sanity by recognizing and identifying false conceptions about our adult children and ourselves. We have begun replacing those destructive lies with spiritually empowering truths.

Over the past few years, God has been showing me how the same SANITY principles (outlined in Part Two of this book) that helped me establish the necessary boundaries regarding my relationship with my son can also be applied to the challenging issues we faced with food and obesity.

The Common Denominator

While there are countless emotional, circumstantial, or even physical reasons why so many people struggle with their weight, there's one common denominator all of us who struggle share—and that, of course, is food itself.

We can "just say no" to enabling our adult children, or allowing difficult people to hurt us. We can put alcohol and other drugs out of our lives—we don't need either substance for survival. Yet it's impossible to "just say no" to food, for without it we would die.

But that doesn't stop us from trying, does it? We try to "just say no" to food by skipping entire meals or going days, weeks, even years in some cases, eating little to nothing, determined to be in control of food and the weight it adds to or subtracts from our bodies. At its worst, this control issue with food can result in life-threatening illnesses such as anorexia, bulimia—or, on the other end of the spectrum, heart attacks, diabetes, and the host of other maladies that can stem from overeating or from eating the wrong foods in excess.

Many of us, in a brave attempt to lose weight, have tried to eat and drink according to some sort of regulated system typically based on two key components: deprivation and reward. In short, in an effort to lose weight we've developed an *unnatural attention on food* while we starve our spirit, soul, mind, and even our body itself of the nourishment it really needs. By dieting, taking pills, using exchange lists and points, and counting calories, fat grams, and carbohydrates, we have been trying to make food behave instead of changing our own behavior.

Setting Boundaries with Food isn't about making food behave; it's about replacing our focus on food with something far more fulfilling. It's about making a series of choices that can free us not only from the pounds that weigh down our bodies, but also from the worry, anxiety, and stress that weigh heavy on our hearts, souls, and spirits. It's about making choices that can bring us into a bountiful relationship with a loving and nurturing God, who can fill the empty places no amount of food can ever reach.

To do this, we must seriously address the emotional and spiritual hunger many of us have ignored. The truth is that we must heal our bodies and souls from the inside out—not from the outside in.

It's from that conviction that I write the books in the Setting Boundaries® series—the conviction that God alone can help us set the necessary boundaries and enable us to make the right choices, bringing us right-side up in whatever issue we're dealing with.

A Reflection of Character

In this fourth book in the Setting Boundaries® series, I'm going to challenge you to give up destructive dieting and unhealthy eating patterns for the last time—to say goodbye to the vicious cycle that has held you prisoner in your own body for years, perhaps even decades.

With so much attention focused on what foods to eat or not to eat, or by ignoring nutrition needs entirely, many of us have stopped paying attention to why we're even eating in the first place.

Are we *really* hungry?

Do our bodies actually need fuel, or are we feeding something else entirely?

The truth is that many of us have never learned how to separate food from feelings. Instead of managing our emotional needs and the internal frustrations related to growth and change, we've fallen into harmful habits of either clinging to food or depriving ourselves of it. We habitually overeat and under eat, habitually watch the numbers on our scale increase and decrease, and habitually start and stop one promising diet after another. When it comes to eating, we've developed many unhealthy and even dangerous habits.

A habit is a pattern of behavior acquired by frequent repetition that reflects the prevailing character of a person. Have you ever thought of your habits as a reflection of your character? As Christians, our character should reflect the character of Christ. We are not born with habits. We develop them—and we can make the choice to change them.

Together, we're going to address the part our emotional needs play in our relationship with food. We're going to see how reorganizing our relationships and understanding our responsibilities can help us set healthy boundaries—boundaries that more deeply reflect the character of Christ. And all the while, we'll be growing spiritually and developing new habits of emotional self-control.

Looking for Love

Many of us have confused the empty space in our stomach with the one in our heart, stuffing one while ignoring the other.

I struggled for decades with my weight as a result of emotional overeating, even for a time becoming morbidly obese. I know what it's like to feel trapped in a seemingly never-ending cycle of dieting, deprivation, despair, and disgust. Weight-related insecurities consumed me for the majority of my life. In fact, there was a time in my twenties when suicide appeared a better option than living another day in an overweight body that I hated. Imagine that—preferring death to being fat.

> My obesity stemmed from boundary-related issues, and my old habit of retreating from emotional pain to the comfort of food was my preferred form of self-medicating. The abuse of food was my attempt to self-soothe and regulate my emotions.

The truth is that the elephant in the room regarding excess weight is our pain and inner emptiness—none of which can be dealt with through fad diets. Some of us, having finally realized the futility of diets that don't address our real hunger, end up treading water from day to day as we desperately try to juggle poor relationships with our loved ones, coworkers, and even with ourselves, due to our poor self-image. We go to sleep at night wondering how we can get through another stressful, boring, unfulfilling, or horrid day. Emotional and physical fatigue has rendered us all but powerless to see the light at the end of the tunnel. In fact, it's often said that many people feel like the light at the end of the tunnel is nothing more than an oncoming train, which is certainly how I felt years ago when my weight soared dangerously close to 300 pounds.

Life-Saving Surgery

For me, as a Christian woman, one answer came as a result of prayer.

Having been diagnosed as morbidly obese, I knew I had to do something to change my life. As I prayed, I decided to look into the admittedly hot-button topic of gastric bypass weight loss surgery. Because it turned out to be a viable starting place for me, I've devoted an entire chapter to this option in this book.

Weight loss surgery (WLS) isn't for everyone, and should never be considered as a panacea for rapid weight loss. While it was an effective tool that helped me lose weight quickly and regain the physical mobility I had lost, it didn't erase the old tapes replaying in my mind, nor did it remove old habits. There are still times when the magnetic pull of the refrigerator is powerful—when food seductively calls my name when I'm not physically hungry. There are times when the trials and tribulations of life seem too big to handle and I find myself being enticed back into my old habits, returning to the false comfort and safety of food.

While I've maintained a 120-pound weight loss for over a decade, the journey to true weight loss freedom came when I discovered the connection between healthy boundaries, spiritual nourishment, and maintaining successful long-term weight loss. Now, I'm keenly aware that my obesity stemmed from boundary-related issues, and my old habit of retreating from emotional pain to the comfort of food was my preferred form of self-medicating. The abuse of food was my attempt to self-soothe and regulate my emotions. Plus, carrying extra weight provided me with a false sense of safety. Protection. It's a good way to keep people at a distance.

When I've told my story, others have confided to me that they have felt the same way. Perhaps you do too. Perhaps you know that your hunger for food is a search for comfort—an attempt to self-medicate the inner emptiness you feel.

I do understand. That's why I'm writing this book. I know from personal experience that it *is* possible to break the cycle of insanity that holds us captive.

My Prayer for You

Today, instead of trying to control my food with the latest fad diet or weight loss trend, I rely on the Six Steps to SANITY that I teach in this book to help me focus on spiritual food. This has sustained me over the years as I've learned more about the role healthy boundaries and balance plays in virtually every aspect of life.

The Six Steps to SANITY can bring hope and healing to hurting hearts. During the course of writing—and living—the Setting Boundaries® books, I've found strength I never knew I had. You can find this strength as well.

> But those who trust in the LORD will find new strength. They will soar high on wings like eagles. They will run and not grow weary. They will walk and not faint (Isaiah 40:31).

This scripture passage has brought me great peace in my journey to set healthy boundaries in many areas of my life and to live the abundant life God has promised. Many of us who deal with the very visible challenge of obesity often have more invisible challenges to overcome. We've spent years hiding behind pounds of pain.

Our lives are incredibly complicated—and often our relationships even more so. As with many of us who find setting boundaries difficult, I came from a fractured family where dysfunctional relationships thrived. I never met my mom's mother, and my dad's mother was a rather taciturn and stoic individual. I don't have many warm and fuzzy grandma memories, but I do remember that she made the best lemon meringue pie. We seldom talked one-on-one, but I vividly recall her words one day when I was a very young girl sitting in her tiny kitchen in Toledo, Ohio. I watched as she added one ingredient and then mixed it in, stopped to add another ingredient, and then mixed some more. Thinking I had come up with a brilliant time-saving option she'd never thought of, I proudly offered some great advice. "Grandma, why don't you just throw everything in the bowl and mix it all at once?" I asked. "That would be easier."

"The easiest way isn't always the right way," Grandma sternly replied, without missing a beat or even looking up to acknowledge me.

That simple exchange was a lesson that stuck with me over the years, and it comes to mind now as I write about the importance of following a progression of six steps on our journey to set healthy boundaries—whether it's with food, adult children, toxic parents, or difficult people.

The right way isn't necessarily going to be the easiest way.

When it comes to confronting issues, breaking habits, and ushering in transformational change that will have lasting implications, there is a right way to find sanity. We already know there's a wrong way—our extra pounds testify to that.

That said, what is the right way—and how do we find it? How do we find sanity in the insane situations and circumstances of life?

It all begins when we reorganize our relationships and understand our responsibilities.

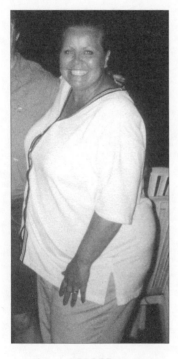

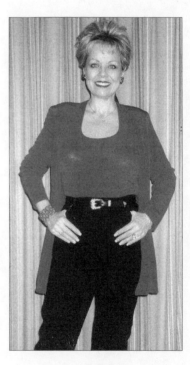

BEFORE	AFTER
My highest weight, close to 300 pounds.	The new me!

Part One

Chapter 1

Reorganizing Our Relationships

My heart stuck in my throat as I looked down at my medical chart. Tears stung my eyes as I tried to comprehend what the doctor had written before excusing himself to take an emergency phone call, leaving my chart lying open on the desk.

Morbidly obese? How dare he!

My initial anger gave way to a deep, incomprehensible pain as the truth of his words sank in. Yes, sometimes truth *is* painful.

I was forty years old and had already resigned myself to going through life being overweight. I seldom got on the scale anymore, oblivious to the numbers that had been ruling my life for so long. But now I had reached the point where I could barely walk up a flight of stairs without gasping for air, and I was seeking medical help. Several years earlier a torn meniscus had required knee surgery. Before that a serious neck injury also required surgery in which a bone graft was inserted into my spine through the front of my throat. Before that, three ruptured disks in my lower back resulted in back surgery, but years later my back still ached. I was in almost constant pain. I was seeing a podiatric surgeon that day to schedule yet another surgery, as bone spurs on my heel were causing excruciating pain with every step. Most physical exercise was nearly impossible. On top of that, I had developed sleep apnea and was having a hard time breathing at night. The fat was literally restricting my airflow when I laid down.

I was falling apart. Carrying around this excess physical baggage was taking a terrible toll. I began to question how it all had happened. *Why can't I control my weight?* I wondered. *What is wrong with me?*

When the doctor returned to the room, I tried valiantly to maintain my composure, as if nothing had happened, and yet my heart was breaking. I fought back tears.

When I got to my car, the floodgates opened.

Crying, I rested my head on the steering wheel as the words "morbidly

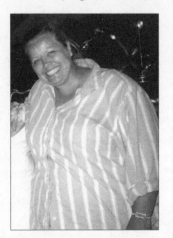

obese" played across my mind's eye like words on an electronic ticker-tape message board. This frightening term meant a lot more than just being overweight.

At this point in my life I really didn't want to starve myself again, which seemed to be the only way I could lose weight—but lately even that didn't work like it had when I was younger. Still, I had to do something. I was so weary of the weight loss dance—lose a few pounds, gain a few more, lose some, gain it back, and around and around I went like the tiny plastic ballerina that spun on the jewelry box I had as a little girl, except at 280 pounds I was anything but little.

"Morbidly obese" was the doctor's devastating diagnosis.

Sitting in my car sobbing, I prayed to God for this dance of dysfunction to end.

Our Unhealthy Relationship with Dieting

The basic premise of most dieting programs is to restrict, reduce, and replace our food intake in some fashion for a specific period of time. Whether it's low-carbohydrate, no-fat, high-protein, all fruit, all vegetables, or liquid only, restrictive diet programs are designed with one primary purpose—to capitalize on our desire (or desperation) to lose weight as quickly as possible—a short-term fix for something that in most cases has been a long-term issue.

Seriously…how many diets have actually worked for you?

Although some weight loss programs may be quite legitimate and healthy, the fact is they keep us focused primarily on food intake, and thus on only one aspect of our lives: the physical.

We'll talk in a later chapter about balancing all aspects of our lives, but it's safe to say that we're comprised of a whole lot more than what we eat and what we weigh, even if the overall goal of most diets seems to ignore this. The Bible clearly points this out: "For life is more than food, and your body more than clothing" (Luke 12:23).

To truly succeed at weight loss, we've got to change the way we think about dieting. We need to find a balance and a sanity that will bring long-term peace and hope to our lives—not just

> Could it be that excess weight is only a symptom, the result of our soul's internal struggle to relinquish control, find love, and experience peace?

short-term weight loss to our bodies. What we need is the strength and determination to stand up and say, "I'm tired of focusing on food and on my weight. This insanity has to stop. Enough is enough!" That cry must be followed by yet another one—this one directed to God as a heartfelt cry to free us from this bondage once and for all.

Confused Priorities and Disordered Relationships

Dieting (as it's practiced by most people who want to lose weight) and setting boundaries with food are two entirely different things. While a focus on the first may or may not yield weight loss, I can almost assure you that a concerted effort to address the second will do so. Returning food to its rightful place in our life can yield amazing results on any number of issues, not the least being our weight. However, it's not easy to set boundaries with food (or with anything for that matter) when we've lost track of where our treasure in life really is, when our priorities are skewed and our relationships are out of kilter. We can change our lives when we change our priorities and re-order our relationships.

Seeing the words "morbidly obese" on my medical chart that day made me take a close look at my priorities and set me on a course for change that led to my passionate study of boundaries and my eventual 120-pound weight loss. But far more importantly, it led to a deeper understanding of what Job meant in the Bible when he said, "I have not departed from his commands, but have treasured his words more than daily food" (Job 23:12).

When there were no more tears to cry in my car that day I dried my eyes, drove home, and got out my dictionary. "Morbid" meant diseased, sickly, unwholesome, grisly, and gruesome. "Obese" meant excessively fat. Suddenly, being overweight took on new meaning—somehow it had metastasized into something far more serious.

How did I get to this place?

Looking Back

I spent the first 35 years of my life entrenched in the New Age movement. For years I jumped from one fad diet to another, from one relationship to another, and from one source of strength and guidance to another. My search for worldly self-actualization left me lost, empty, and hopeless. With an unnatural and unhealthy focus on food, I lost and regained hundreds of pounds during those years.

Then I came to a point in my life where my spiritual quest turned from the emptiness of the New Age movement to the fullness of a Christian experience with Christ as my Lord. And although that brought about the spiritual change I had been seeking, my struggles with food and weight didn't magically disappear when I asked the Lord into my life. It wasn't a "find faith and lose weight" two-step program. You see, faith requires a response to God's commandments, and God's most important commandment is that we love Him, that we have a relationship with Him, that we relinquish the control of our life and yield everything to Him.

> We can change our lives when we change our priorities and re-order our relationships.

Yielding is all about faith and trust—do we take matters into our own hands and try to fill our own needs (or perceived needs), or do we entrust these needs to God as our heavenly Father and provider? I had to ask the question: Is there an unmet need in my life that causes me to turn to food for fulfillment instead of turning to God?

Matthew 16:25 says, "If you try to hang on to your life, you will lose it. But if you give up your life for my sake, you will save it." Could it be that excess weight is only a symptom, the result of our soul's internal struggle to relinquish control, find love, and experience peace?

When it comes to setting healthy boundaries, I've learned it's usually about control—losing it, gaining it, maintaining it, and understanding who really has it to begin with. It took me years to fully comprehend the vital truth that God is in control, my body belongs to Him, and there is a level of stewardship required of me concerning this earthly vessel He has entrusted to my care.

> Don't you realize that your body is the temple of the Holy Spirit, who lives in you and was given to you by God? You do not belong to yourself, for God bought you with a high price. So you must honor God with your body (1 Corinthians 6:19-20).

I'd read that scripture numerous times but somehow always managed to glide over it. I never thought of my weight as dishonoring to God until the words "morbidly obese" entered the picture, ushering in a landslide of scriptural revelation and spiritual conviction that would utterly change my life.

As the great writer Oswald Chambers said, "Christianity is not walking in the light of our convictions but walking in the light of the Lord, a very different thing. Convictions are necessary, but only as stepping stones to all that God wants us to be."[1]

God wants us to be more than what we eat—or weigh.

God Will Reveal Himself

As a relatively new believer I was still navigating the terrain of faith, trying to figure out God's plan and purpose for my life. Newly remarried and living in the Midwest, I was happy in my personal life, my writing career looked hopeful as I'd just secured my first literary agent, and I'd convinced myself that, comparatively speaking, my emotional health was the best it had ever been. Life was good—if you didn't take into consideration that my weight was increasing every year, that physically my body was a wreck, and that I'd just been listed on my medical chart as "morbidly obese."

I hadn't spent much time focusing on what God wanted me to be. I felt certain I knew what God wanted me to *do* with my life (write) but insofar as knowing all He wanted me to *be*, I wasn't sure.

When it came right down to it I had the human *doing* thing mastered—but reaching the human *being* stage took me considerably longer. My thinking was still so scrambled from decades of painful memories, poor choices, and something I didn't want to admit even to myself—a profound lack of trust that I was really safe in the arms of God.

I love what author Henry Blackaby writes about this kind of mixed-up thinking in his acclaimed book *Experiencing God*:

> When your life is in the middle of God's activity, He will start rearranging a lot of your thinking. God's ways and thoughts are so different from yours and mine that they will often sound wrong, crazy, or impossible. Often, you will realize that the task is far beyond your power or resources to accomplish. When you recognize that the task is humanly impossible, you need to be ready to believe God and trust Him completely.
>
> You need to believe that He will enable and equip you to do everything He asks of you. Don't try to second-guess Him. Just let Him be God. Turn to Him for the needed power, insight, skill, and resources. He will provide you with all you need.[2]

What I needed was to stop worrying about how I got to this place of morbid obesity and concentrate on how I was going to get out, starting with asking God to rearrange my "stinkin' thinkin'." I needed to get a handle on this weight issue for the last time, and I couldn't do it alone.

Putting Food in Its Rightful Place

One of the first things God provided was a new perspective about food. I'd been obsessed with it for all of my adult life, and I tried to control it so I could lose weight quickly. I'd been on every diet program imaginable. Just as Henry Blackaby had written, God began to rearrange my thinking, starting with His Word. He began to reveal fresh insight to me through Bible study and research.

Food is mentioned 349 times in the New Living Translation and 373 times in the New International Version. The references range from the literal interpretation of Genesis 1:29 where God said, "Look! I have given you every seed-bearing plant throughout the earth and all the fruit trees for your food" to the more spiritual interpretations: "'My food,' said Jesus, 'is to do the will of him who sent me and to finish his work'" (John 4:34 NIV).

Intended by God to nourish our physical body, food now plays numerous roles in our life, and unfortunately not all of them are healthy. Many of us have spent a lifetime trying to control the food we eat...or don't eat. Dieting isn't something we occasionally do—it's how we've learned to live. We are obsessed with and consumed by food. In fact, our relationship with food has become one of the most important relationships we have.

And that misplaced focus makes the Enemy very happy indeed.

One of Satan's most successful strategies to attack and influence the children of God has been to keep them too involved with challenging relationships to care about a relationship with the One who cares the most— Jesus Christ—and for many of us the most challenging relationship we have is the one we have with food. Food is dependable and available when we need it. Food doesn't leave, talk back, or have a mind of its own. Food doesn't judge. Food is our comforter and confidant, demanding nothing of us. Food represents safety, trust, and love. Food can keep us alive or contribute to our demise. Food has become our friend, enemy, lover, and abuser all rolled into one.

Could there be a more challenging, or—dare I say it?—dysfunctional relationship?

Imagine all we could do if we returned food to its rightful place in our lives. Imagine what would happen if we could see with absolute clarity how clever Satan has been in his quest to divert us from the truth that our magnificent obsession was never intended to be a relationship with food—but instead with the One who provides it.

Our Most Important Relationship

Setting Boundaries with Food is about taking responsibility for our lives and our choices, including the choice to intentionally develop and nurture the important relationships that define who we are—relationships with ourselves, others, food, and most important, with God.

God wants us to finish the work He has called us to do, to be the people He created us to be, and to live purposeful and productive lives. He wants to rain down tremendous blessings on our lives, to abundantly provide all we could ever hope for. He wants to answer every prayer of every faithful heart. In return, He wants our most important relationship to be with Him—for our magnificent obsession to be *Him*.

But that's difficult to do when our relationships are all tangled up and we're confused about our priorities and our responsibilities. In their book *Daily Disciples*, authors David Wardell and Jeff Leever impart a simple but powerful truth:

> In the Christian journey through life, I believe we're either moving closer to God every day, or we're moving away from Him. The choice is ours. We all have a responsibility to grow in Christ. We can't—*you can't*—afford to ignore the longing of our souls...that sense that we need to be closer to Him.[3]

Could it be many of us are ignoring the "longing of our souls"? Could this be why we have an unhealthy focus on food, eating, dieting, and weight?

When it comes to priorities, God sets some very clear boundaries and standards for how He wants us to live.

> Jesus replied, "'You must love the LORD your God with all your heart, all your soul, and all your mind.' This is the first and greatest commandment. A second is equally important: 'Love your neighbor as yourself.' The entire law and all the demands of the prophets are based on these two commandments" (Matthew 22:37-40).

Relationships are a necessary part of healthy living, but there is no such thing as a perfect relationship between human beings. Relationships, from friendships to romances, are mercurial and have the potential to take us from the highest of highs to the lowest of lows. There is only one relationship in which we can experience perfect truth: our relationship with God.

Because of His love for us, His will for us is always best. Because of His power, there are things only He can do in our lives. When we make knowing Him our number-one priority our lives can profoundly change, as Henry Blackaby writes:

> Knowing God does not come through a program, a study, or a method. It is the result of a vibrant, growing, one-on-one relationship with God. Within this intimate connection, God will reveal Himself, His purposes, and His ways so you can know Him in deeper and profound dimensions. As you relate to Him, God will invite you to join in His activity where He is already at work. When you obey, God accomplishes through you things only He can do. As the Lord works in and through your life, you will come to know Him ever more closely.[4]

Recently, I watched on TV the creation of a ten-layer birthday cake, each layer representing ten years of life. Alternating five-inch layers of chocolate and vanilla cake with one-inch layers of buttercream frosting, this was a five-foot-tall masterpiece with an icing of fondant painted to look like moiré taffeta in a shade of robin's egg blue. It was all rather stupendous to behold, and yet the real key to its success was the three-inch-wide PVC post running through the center and anchoring the layers together. The post was unseen by anyone looking at the beautiful creation, yet without this core foundation the cake could never have stood upright. The layers would most certainly have slid off of each other and onto the floor.

Our relationship with God is the strength in our center, keeping the layers of our lives from falling to pieces around us.

Reorganizing Our Relationships

For many of us who struggle with weight issues, our relationship with food is like the adult child who breaks our heart, the toxic aging parent whose needs are increasing, or the difficult person who pushes our buttons. Food has become the dysfunctional relationship with which we have developed an unhealthy dependence, and it's time for us to break up the romance.

Author Anne Katherine expounds on our unhealthy connection with food.

> To some small extent, almost everyone is dependent on food for relief of more than hunger. Food is used for many purposes other than nutritional survival. It is used to soften people up socially, to sell houses, to manipulate business sales, to impress a date, as a centerpiece for activities, to stabilize families, to unite a culture. In fact, food is probably used for psychological purposes more than any other activity or substance.
>
> For some of us, however, food is like a lifeline, an essential tool in our emotional survival kit. It takes us away from stress, it numbs our fears and worries, and it stops the world and lets us get off. It's a womb, a haven, a cave, an escape, and a refuge.
>
> Eating is an automatic response to feelings—so quickly applied without thought—that breaking this pattern takes tremendous sustained effort. To diminish the power of the bond with food takes a revolution. If food has become a cornerstone, and the cornerstone is to be removed, an equally strong foundation must replace it.[5]

I've discovered something as I've grown in my walk as a child of God. He opens my eyes and heart in direct proportion to how much I open my arms to Him. When I put my relationship with Him in a priority perspective, and understand what is and isn't my responsibility, life seems to flow much better. While this sounds relatively easy, it requires a concerted effort to develop positive habits that foster intentional and deliberate life choices. But with God all things truly are possible.

It's time for us to nurture healthy relationships that will replace the dysfunctional ones we have with food—starting with the pivotal relationship that will be the foundational cornerstone needed to transform all of the relationships in our lives. Our relationship with God is intended to nourish our spirits, souls, hearts, and minds. Food is intended to nourish our bodies.

Healthy Relationships

A healthy relationship enriches our lives and adds to our enjoyment of life. Life can be filled with joy and promise when two people develop a connection based on healthy characteristics such as mutual respect, trust, honesty, support, fairness and equality, separate identities, good communication, and a sense of playfulness and fondness.

Every relationship is a combination of both healthy and unhealthy characteristics. This applies to all relationships: work relationships, friendships, family, and romantic relationships. However, a healthy relationship should bring more happiness than stress into your life. Every relationship will have stress at times, but prolonged mental stress on either member is not a sign of a healthy relationship.

Unhealthy Relationships

Unhealthy relationships exhibit characteristics that cause stress and pressure. This tension can include physical or verbal abuse, manipulation, anger, control, criticism, or lack of respect. Are you drawn to a particular type of friend, job, or perhaps even a hobby—someone or something—that never fails to have a negative impact on your life? Is there an unhealthy relationship or habit you can't seem to break away from that has brought prolonged mental stress and often leaves you broken and bruised, seeking comfort in the warm embrace of food?

Challenging Relationships

Sometimes, sad to say, the relationships we have with people bring us far less pleasure than the delight we get from a plate of crispy fries, a bag of crunchy potato chips, or a pint of rich and creamy ice cream. In fact, sometimes the relationships we have with challenging people are contributing factors when we turn to food for comfort. Unfortunately, crazy-making relationships can keep us in bondage for years.

Perhaps you've heard of this definition of insanity. It's "repeating the same behavior and expecting different results." Let me tell you, I was the Queen

> God opens our eyes and heart in direct proportion to how much we open our arms to Him.

of Insanity for more years than I care to remember. How about you? Do you have people in your life who never fail to push your buttons and rub your nerves raw? Have you repeated the same actions over and over again, expecting different results? Now, think about your relationship with food in that same context. Have you lost and regained the same 20, 40, or 60 pounds over and over again?

If you're repeating the same dieting behavior and expecting different results, chances are there's a lot more insanity going on in your life than meets the eye.

Don't lose heart—sanity is possible! But we must be willing to change the habits that keep us on a perpetual gerbil wheel—going around and around with no end in sight.

> We've got to get to the bottom of what's eating us for us to seriously change why we're eating.

June Hunt is the founder of Hope for the Heart, a worldwide biblical counseling ministry that, for more than 20 years, has provided a wide variety of resources for people seeking answers. She hosts a live two-hour call-in counseling program called Hope in the Night and has authored numerous books. In her book *How to Rise Above Abuse*, June identifies the key characteristics of healthy and unhealthy relationships:

> Are you in an abusive relationship? Have you experienced an unhealthy dynamic between you and someone close to you? Many people fail to recognize that they are in an abusive relationship because abuse has been "their normal" for so long. If you look closely, you can evaluate the health of any relationship by seeing the type of fruit it produces—whether the fruit is good or bad. Jesus said, "A good tree cannot bear bad fruit, and a bad tree cannot bear good fruit. Every tree that does not bear good fruit is cut down and thrown into the fire. Thus, by their fruit you will recognize them" (Matthew 7:18-20 NIV).[6]

Henry Blackaby agrees. "If you are experiencing a time of fruitlessness right now," he writes, "you may be trying to do things on your own that God has not initiated."[7]

When we look at our relationship with food through this lens of fruitlessness and abuse, is it any wonder we've struggled for so long? Many of us have been in abusive relationships with food for years, bearing nothing but bad fruit, and we don't even know it.

Removing the Blinders

We've got to get to the bottom of what's eating us for us to seriously change why we're eating. Could it be the reason many of us avoid addressing painful or traumatic life issues is because we've spent years stuffing them as far down as possible and we don't want to dredge up the truth? Could it be that it's easier now to create our own truth, evading the deep heart issues at the core of who we are, affecting everything we say and do?

I was morbidly obese because I'd abused my body for years with improper nutrition, destructive diets, and a lack of physical exercise. I had never learned how to set healthy boundaries—not only with food, but in most of my significant relationships, including my relationship with my adult son. I was so busy taking care of other people, things, and business, that I didn't have time (or make time) to focus on my responsibility to treat my body as a temple of the Holy Spirit. I was morbidly obese as a result of living years in emotional turmoil and frequently stuffing the empty hole in my soul with food. I was morbidly obese because my life was grossly out of balance—and when all was said and done, I had only myself to blame. Sure, there were genetic factors and body chemistry issues at play, but a time came when I could no longer justify my weight and ignore my health.

God began to seriously convict me that I was responsible for the choices I was making. I hadn't been making very good ones, and if I didn't jump off this train now while I still could, it would soon be too late. It was increasing speed, heading for a destination of destruction. Time was up. I had to reorganize my relationships, understand my responsibilities, and begin to set healthy boundaries. But I knew I needed help on the journey. I couldn't be objective on my own.

Therapeutic Relationships

When I began my relationship with the Lord I had a son addicted to heroin. He was in jail more often than he was out. At first, I isolated this situation from others, believing (wrongly) that good Christian parents didn't have children who were involved in drugs and crime. I believed I would be judged harshly if anyone knew the extent of the truth. In time, I came to understand that this was not the case.

It's important to not isolate yourself during any time of emotional, spiritual, and physical change, regardless of what you may be dealing with. We were created to be in relationship with God the Father and with other brothers and sisters in Christ. There is nothing to be ashamed of if you feel the need to seek out a support group or talk with a professional counselor or psychologist to get your life back on track. In fact, it could be the best call you ever make.

It was surely the best call I ever made, on several occasions, and I can say without hesitation that it's by the grace of God and the direction of gifted counselors that I've been able to traverse some seemingly impossible obstacles over the years.

Professional therapy might be the best way to go when we need to make significant changes in our life. Having the benefit of an objective opinion and the therapeutic advice of a professional is invaluable. In addition to professional counseling, there are many resources available to us at little or no cost. We may have to conduct a bit of research to find them, but it will be worth it. For many of us, it's much too difficult to heal without objective, qualified, and nonjudgmental help.

Charting Our Course

As we move on in this book, there are some things I want you to do that will help you incorporate its message.

I would hazard a guess that at one point or another in your weight loss journey you've written down the foods you've eaten, the times you've eaten, the calories you've consumed, the exchange points used, or the numbers on the scale.

This time, let's take a different route.

As we navigate this new path to sanity, let's consider ourselves modern day cartographers as we commit to recording the terrain of our lives on paper. Please get a spiral notebook, blank journal, or pad of paper that will fit easily into your purse, briefcase, or carryall bag. I'll be giving you writing assignments throughout this book, and I hope you'll choose to complete them.

It was during counseling for my own boundary and weight-related issues years ago that I first learned the value of recording and journaling my thoughts, memories, and feelings. It's an integral part of this book today not only because it was an integral part of my ability to find freedom from the bondage of dieting and food obsession, but it has been proven beneficial in numerous therapeutic environments.

As you begin to write, you will notice a budding clarity emerging. Without this process your thoughts would likely stay jumbled up inside your head. Write whatever comes to mind first—there are no right or wrong answers. The goal is not to write perfect prose, but to prime the pump of your memory. Do your best not to censor yourself. No one will see this but you (unless you choose to share it).

The power of putting pen to paper can begin to take on a life of its own—even for those who don't typically write. The more you write, the deeper you will go into places you've long forgotten or perhaps didn't even believe existed. For some of us the memories will be vivid. For others they may be hard to retrieve—and even harder to record on paper. But press on. Don't give up.

Please understand I'm not insinuating that everyone who is struggling with boundary issues concerning food has been a victim of abuse. I'm sure that isn't the case. However, if you have been dealing with overeating, compulsive eating, or yo-yo dieting for more than a few years, I pray you will keep an open mind concerning the possibility that you may be using food as a way to stuff down emotions or memories that you'd rather not deal with, feelings that may trigger an emotional reaction.

It's also important to be aware that God really does work in mysterious ways, and there are no accidents in His Kingdom. You're holding this book right now for a very specific purpose, whether it's to change your life or to be a change agent in the life of someone else. There are powerful forces at work all around us.

In *Experiencing God*, Henry Blackaby pulls no punches in warning readers to be prepared for major adjustments when implementing any kind of change that involves our relationship with God. As he says, "You cannot stay where you are and go with God at the same time."[8] As you embark on this journey to find sanity in a life that may be anything but sane at the moment, my prayer is that in addition to keeping your eyes wide open you will also open your heart in even greater measure, giving God full reign to do what only He can do in your life.

A New Perspective

Our first responsibility is to make our relationship with God the most important in our lives—to trust, obey, and depend entirely on Him.

If you find that difficult to do, pray for God to show you how to love Him in real, personal, and practical ways. Ask Him to reveal His love, grace, mercy, and power to you. God wants to pursue a deeply meaningful love relationship with us, and He can enable us to accomplish His will. He is completely able to free us from the bondage of any relationship that breaks our hearts or keeps us distanced from Him.

Are you ready for Him to do that?

Take time now to write in your journal about your relationship with God.

1. How would you describe your relationship with God?

2. How would you like this relationship to look in the future?

3. What is God revealing to you about unhealthy relationships?

4. What new directions is God showing you for developing healthy relationships?

5. Have you ever thought of food and eating in the context of being in a relationship with them?

In his letter to the church in Corinth, the apostle Paul speaks of our "fearful responsibility" to being accountable to what we have done with our lives as Christians.

> Because we understand our fearful responsibility to the Lord, we work hard to persuade others. God knows we are sincere, and I hope you know this, too (2 Corinthians 5:11).

Reorganizing our relationships is the beginning of taking fearful responsibility for our actions and living a life of purpose that is pleasing to God.

Chapter 2

Understanding Our Responsibilities

I've talked with hundreds of women and men around the world about the topic of boundaries. It's clear that not only do many of us lack healthy relationship priorities, but we're confused and often deeply troubled about what *is* and *isn't* our responsibility in our relationships. As a result, we tend to respond to the ensuing havoc in sometimes catastrophically unhealthy ways.

Very early in my journey of trying to better understand God's plan for my life, there was a pivotal book that gave me biblical insight into the world of intangible boundaries—the boundaries that define who we are at the core of our being. Written by Henry Cloud and John Townsend, *Boundaries: When to Say Yes, When to Say No to Take Control of Your Life* is the benchmark resource for Christians who desire to gain insight into the destructive patterns that keep people dysfunctional. Here is the authors' perspective on the issue of responsibility.

> Made in the image of God, we were created to take responsibility for certain tasks. Part of taking responsibility, or ownership, is in knowing what *is* our job, and what *isn't*. Workers who continually take on duties that aren't theirs will eventually burn out. It takes wisdom to know what we should be doing and what we shouldn't. We can't do everything.[1]

We Can't Do It All

I've had many friends over the years who struggled with being overweight. I can tell you firsthand they were seldom sitting on the sofa eating chips and watching TV, as is the caricature of overweight people. Quite the opposite, in fact. These are some of the busiest people I have known, in many instances biting off far more than they could chew (no pun intended) in their desire to help in whatever way possible. It's no accident that many of us dealing with weight-related issues have spent years trying to "do everything"…except take care of the bodies God has given us.

Making healthy choices that balance our own needs with the needs of others rests on our own shoulders. In making the changes that will affect our attitude toward food, we can—and must—also make significant changes in how we view our responsibilities to ourselves, to others, and to God.

A Hierarchy of Responsibility

There are countless illustrations I could share about the good intentions of well-meaning men and women who truly desire to help the people they care about, but have taken on responsibilities that weren't theirs in the first place and have neglected their own responsibilities in the process.

Are you one of those well-intentioned souls?

If so, the time has come to re-order your responsibilities. This is the order in which our relationships and responsibilities should fall:

Our Relationship with…	Our Responsibility to…
God	God
Ourselves	Ourselves
Others	Others
Food	Food

Assuming Responsibility

One of the reasons *Setting Boundaries with Your Adult Children* has been so helpful to a great many parents is because it redirects personal responsibility to where it should be…even if that redirection is, at first, painful. As I wrote in that book,

Although it's high time many of our adult children begin to

accept the consequences of their choices, the plain truth is that *we must first accept the responsibility for our choices*—past choices, present choices, and future choices.

Our biggest problem isn't our adult children's inability to wake up when their alarm clocks ring, or their inability to keep a schedule, or their inability to hold down jobs or pay their bills. It's not their drug use or alcohol addictions. It's not the mess they're making of their lives. The main problem is the part we're playing in stepping in to soften the blow of the consequences that come from the choices they make.

The main problem is us.

Ouch.[2]

When I wrote that I knew I was being hard on parents, but I felt convicted that someone had to be hard, and who better than a fellow parent in pain? Once I understood my part in enabling my adult son, it wasn't difficult to see that I needed to implement healthy boundaries and find sanity. And it all began when the doctor declared me "morbidly obese." It was a catalyst that motivated me to make new choices to change.

What is it that has motivated you to consider making a change?

Today, thousands of parents and grandparents have experienced newfound freedom and sanity in their relationships with adult children, and I would hazard a guess a great many adult children have been faced with finally accepting the consequences of their choices—or not. My desire wasn't to throw a generation of adult kids under the bus, but to empower parents and grandparents to step back and actually allow their adult children to board the bus—on their own—and to take responsibility for their own choices. I've been encouraging parents for years to take the spotlight off our adult children and shine it on ourselves instead. It's a hard pill for some of us to swallow. It's not easy to look at the part we have played, not in *causing* the problems, but in how we've *responded* to the problems.

Likewise, food isn't causing our problems. It's how we use and abuse food in responding to our problems.

The Real Issue

Our biggest problem isn't that our boss has unreasonable expectations, or that our ex-spouse refuses to abide by the rules outlined in the divorce decree. It's not that some of our loved ones are addicted to drugs or alcohol, or about the mess they're making of their lives. It's not the fault of fast-food restaurants or million-dollar advertising campaigns or the never-ending stream of diets that don't work. It's not about any of the things we've been using as reasons for overeating.

If we have a problem in our relationship with food, the main problem isn't the food. The main problem is how we relate to food—how we use food as an anesthetic to dull our feelings.

Once again, the main problem is us.

And once again I say, ouch.

Our Responsibility to God

In her book *No Limits No Boundaries*, Pastor Tiz Huch doesn't imply that we don't need boundaries, but that when we enter into right relationship with God, His love, grace, mercy, and forgiveness have no end. When we act as children of God we have choices to make, and those choices should revolve around how God wants us to act. He has established boundaries as written in Scripture, and He has instructed us to live according to them. As Pastor Tiz puts it,

> God has put you in the place where you are, at this particular time, for a specific purpose! However, not everyone responds to this call. The few who are chosen are the ones who answer the call and accept God's offer. God makes His move; then the ball is in our court! It's up to us to respond in faith by accepting Christ in our hearts and acting as His children. In doing this, we become the "chosen ones." With this freedom of choice, though, comes the option of ignoring God's invitation and thereby being excluded from the "chosen ones." I don't want this to sound ominous, but the truth is that our futures are determined by the choices we make. Many people don't want to take responsibility for their futures. It's much easier just to hang out, hang on, and hope for the best. We need to realize that today's decisions determine tomorrow's destiny![3]

Having rich, fertile soil from which our choices can grow and bear fruit is important. In *How to Rise Above Abuse*, June Hunt writes about having personal standards for Christian living.

> Within the boundaries of biblical absolutes, God gives us the responsibility to choose how we will live our Christian lives. The choices we make throughout the day as to how we will present ourselves to others and how we will conduct ourselves around others reflect our standards. *Making choices* to live by biblical standards is not legalism, even if the choices we make are more conservative or restrictive than the choices of others…We need to submit to God's authority; we are accountable to God first and to human authority second.[4]

A Mandate from God

We guard our personal property with fences, locked doors, and elaborate security systems. We guard our money in banks, safety deposit boxes, and vaults. Sports enthusiasts guard their bodies with helmets, padded uniforms, and mouthpieces. But even with an ever-increasing focus on guarding what is important to us, when it comes to our most valuable asset we are sorely deficient in accepting responsibility.

Solomon tells us, "Above all else, guard your heart, for everything you do flows from it" (Proverbs 4:23 NIV). We are responsible for guarding our hearts, and we guard our hearts by establishing healthy boundaries around them. These boundaries includes balancing our needs with the needs of others.

Our Responsibility to Ourselves

Contrary to politically correct opinion, we're not all created equal, especially when it comes to needs.

Yes, there are some needs that everyone shares, such as oxygen, water, and, yes, food. We all need those things to survive—that's a given. However, it's the more personal needs that often trip us up—the individualized needs that set us apart from others. Such needs are not categorically wrong or right—just different. For example, I'm extremely uncomfortable in dark rooms. I need a source of illumination in a room to feel safe. You may not have that same need, but that doesn't diminish the validity it carries in my life. But it's my responsibility to address this need in my life.

Making choices that balance our own needs with the needs of others isn't always easy. It's difficult to guard our hearts and maintain personal boundaries in life when we're being pressed on all sides by countless tasks as our own needs are shuffled down on the list. And therein lays the crux of this entire issue of setting healthy boundaries—identifying and addressing our needs. A great many things vie for our attention—and there are only so many hours in a day.

Something has to give.

Often, it's our sanity.

But it's okay if our needs aren't being addressed, right? After all, our goal as good Christians is to serve others and put ourselves aside, right? Being a good Christian is all about sacrifice and dying to self, right? If our responsibilities for others in our lives are already consuming the majority of our time, what does it say about us if we put on the brakes and stop long enough to take care of our own needs—if we set boundaries in our relationships? That we're selfish and self-centered, that we're bad Christians, right?

Wrong. Nothing could be farther from the truth.

It's important to our heavenly Father that we guard our hearts and grow in a healthy heart relationship with Him. He never intended for us to be responsible for everyone except ourselves. The more time we spend in His presence, asking Him to order our steps, the more clarity we will have on our responsibilities.

In *One-Minute Prayers for Women*, Hope Lyda speaks to this issue of responsibility.

> God, let me dive into the tasks I have before me at work and at home. I want to face my responsibilities with great strength and effort. I want to be hard working in every setting. May my focus be to serve You, no matter what the job. When I honor You with the labor of my hands and mind, I know that strengthens me spiritually. Everything is connected to what is good and right. Lead me to responsibilities that are

of importance to you. Guide me away from fruitless efforts. I want my life to count. I want my work to please You.[5]

Is our work pleasing to God? Or are we overwhelmed with the burdens of too much responsibility? How can we keep Him as the priority relationship in our lives and be responsible for ourselves as well as for those He has placed in our lives?

Reflect on these questions in your journal, praying for fresh insight from God.

Our One-Day-at-a-Time Responsibility

If we truly want to balance our responsibilities and build healthy relationships, we must become emotionally strong and take control of the things we *can* control. The well-known Serenity Prayer is good to remember at this time. The Serenity Prayer is the common name for an originally untitled prayer by the theologian Reinhold Niebuhr, and has been adopted by Alcoholics Anonymous and other twelve-step programs.

> God grant me the serenity to accept the things I cannot change; courage to change the things I can; and wisdom to know the difference.

Accepting what we cannot change is understanding what is and isn't our responsibility. Having the courage to change what we can is accepting our responsibility and taking action. In some cases that will mean setting boundaries. Ask God to direct your path and give you wisdom and clear discernment concerning the direction you should take.

Historical documentation available on the origination of A.A.'s use of the phrase "One day at a time" indicates an overall "origin unknown" status. However, I'd like to believe it comes directly from Scripture. Over the years a host of support groups around the world have adopted the phrase and there's a scripturally sound reason for that. It's God's plan for how He wants us to live. Taken from the book of Matthew, the meaning is crystal clear:

> That is why I tell you not to worry about everyday life—whether you have enough food and drink, or enough clothes

to wear. Isn't life more than food, and your body more than clothing? Look at the birds. They don't plant or harvest or store food in barns, for your heavenly Father feeds them. And aren't you far more valuable to him than they are? Can all your worries add a single moment to your life?

And why worry about your clothing? Look at the lilies of the field and how they grow. They don't work or make their clothing, yet Solomon in all his glory was not dressed as beautifully as they are. And if God cares so wonderfully for wildflowers that are here today and thrown into the fire tomorrow, he will certainly care for you. Why do you have so little faith?

So don't worry about these things, saying, "What will we eat? What will we drink? What will we wear?" These things dominate the thoughts of unbelievers, but your heavenly Father already knows all your needs. Seek the Kingdom of God above all else, and live righteously, and he will give you everything you need.

So don't worry about tomorrow, for tomorrow will bring its own worries. Today's trouble is enough for today (Matthew 6:25-34).

In other words, take it "one day at a time."

Getting Back on Track

This problem of being overly responsible is becoming an epidemic. We're not sure anymore what's really normal, what a boundary is or isn't, what we're actually supposed to be responsible for, or even what it means to live a balanced life. The only way we're going to be able to sort any of this out is to explore how and when our lives started to go haywire in the first place.

How did our relationships and responsibilities get so off track and our lives become so unmanageable that we turned to food as the answer?

Two words: *unhealthy boundaries.*

Chapter 3

Defining Our Boundaries

I craned my neck to try to see around the cars lined up in front of me as we approached one of the busiest intersections in my city. Was it an accident that had traffic moving at a snail's pace? Glancing up, I noticed the signal lights were all flashing red, including those directing the two left-turn lanes at all four points.

It became clear as cars moved forward that either some folks didn't know the "person on the right goes first" rule or this sudden change in routine had caused momentary amnesia. Some people ignored the traffic rule, the painted boundary lines, and all sense of civilized decorum as well, crossing haphazardly into other lanes, laying on horns, yelling out of windows, and gesturing wildly. It was utter havoc!

We need structure, especially when we come together publicly in groups. Without an understanding of the structure provided by boundaries—and a willingness to respect them—things can get complicated, overwhelming, and dangerous. In most cases, boundaries can be blessings!

Visible boundaries such as fences, signs, and dividing lines painted on streets and highways are easy to identify, but boundaries can also be unseen, invisible structures that support healthy, productive lives. These invisible boundaries can sometimes be more difficult to identify.

Unseen—not *nonexistent*.

There's a big difference.

What Is a Boundary?

Webster defines a boundary as "something that marks or fixes a limit... a territory, border, frontier."

The most recognizable boundaries are property lines. No Trespassing signs posted on private property send a clear message: If you cross the line you will be prosecuted! This type of physical boundary is easy to understand because it's tangible; you can actually see and touch the sign. On the other hand, personal boundaries are harder to define because the lines are invisible. Also, they can change and they are unique to each individual.

Why We Need Boundaries

On our journey to make healthy choices that will change our lives, one of the first things we must learn is why we need boundaries in the first place. Quite simply, we need them because God has mandated them. This is the way He wants us to live. God set the first boundary in the Garden of Eden.

> The LORD God took the man and put him in the Garden of Eden to work it and take care of it. And the LORD God commanded the man, "You are free to eat from any tree in the garden; but you must not eat from the tree of the knowledge of good and evil, for when you eat from it you will certainly die" (Genesis 2:15-17 NIV).

As we know, Adam and Eve overstepped this boundary. The consequences were catastrophic.

The most basic boundary-setting word is *no* (as in, "No, I'd rather not have another piece of pie" or "No, I'm unable to work your shift for you today as I've already made other plans"). It lets others know that you exist apart from them and that you are in control of you. Being clear about your no—and your yes—is a theme that runs throughout the Bible.

> All you need to say is simply "Yes" or "No"; anything beyond this comes from the evil one (Matthew 5:37 NIV).

> Above all, my brothers and sisters, do not swear—not by heaven or by earth or by anything else. All you need to say is a simple "Yes" or "No." Otherwise you will be condemned (James 5:12 NIV).

Boundaries and Selfishness

Unfortunately, people often view boundaries negatively, especially Christians, as if setting boundaries were just an excuse to reject others or be selfish.

Nothing could be farther from the truth, as the authors share in their seminal book *Boundaries: When to Say Yes, When to Say No to Take Control of Your Life.*

> For years, Christians have been taught that protecting their spiritual and emotional property is selfish. Yet God is interested in people loving others, and you can't love others unless you have received love inside yourself.
>
> This principle is illustrated when the psalmist says, "above all else, guard your heart, for everything you do flows from it" (Proverbs 4:23 NIV). When we "watch over" our hearts (the home of our treasures), we guard them.[1]

Boundaries and Emotional Choices

Another reason we have trouble setting boundaries, and one of the most prevalent, is that we're too emotionally involved in situations to consider them objectively. In such cases, we often rely on our feelings rather than thinking the matter through. When possible, our choices should be made calmly, rationally, and with prayerful wisdom, especially when they significantly affect our relationships. Unfortunately, that's much easier said than done and it's impossible for many of us to accomplish without the divine grace and guidance of God.

When it comes to emotions, many of us are like gerbils on a wheel—going around and around, out of control and seemingly unable to stop the habits we've developed. We do this because:

- We don't think we have a choice.
- We've neglected to define our personal boundaries.
- Our own destructive patterns get in the way.
- We've lost sight of our priorities.

- We don't understand our identity, our place within the family of God.

Unfortunately, the habits we've developed to address emotional situations and circumstances often include numerous trips to the refrigerator, pantry, or vending machine, just to get "a little something" to take the edge off the moment.

The Freedom of Boundaries

Boundaries can bring freedom into your life and into the life of your relationships. But we must know what a boundary is and what it isn't. We've already defined a boundary, but let's consider the definition in contrast with what it is not. Although this seems like basic information, it's important that we change the old tapes that still play inside our brain, telling us lies about boundaries that Satan has successfully used to keep us in bondage.

What a Boundary Is:	What a Boundary Is Not:
Healthy	Rejection
Necessary	Selfish
Biblical	Sinful
Respectful	Disrespectful
Loving	Dishonoring

Types of Boundaries

Personal boundary lines define who we are and influence all areas of our lives. Most of us are so concerned about our overwhelming responsibilities that we don't recognize the intangible boundaries that define many facets of our daily lives. We need to recognize that we have boundaries in many areas, including personal boundaries, physical boundaries, psychological boundaries (also known as emotional or intellectual boundaries), and spiritual boundaries. Let's examine each in turn.

Personal Boundaries

Personal boundaries are limits or borders that define where you end and others begin. Your personal boundary is defined by the amount of physical and emotional space you allow between yourself and others. Personal boundaries also help you decide what types of communication, behavior, and interaction you accept from others. The types of boundaries you set defines whether you have healthy or unhealthy relationships.

I like the way Henry Cloud and John Townsend clarify this:

> Any confusion of responsibility and ownership in our lives is a problem of boundaries. Just as homeowners set physical property lines around their land, we need to set mental, physical, emotional, and spiritual boundaries around our heart, to help us distinguish what is our responsibility and what isn't. The inability to set appropriate boundaries at appropriate times with the appropriate people can be very destructive. And this is one of the most serious problems facing Christians today. Many sincere, dedicated believers struggle with tremendous confusion about when it is biblically appropriate to set limits.[2]

Physical Boundaries

Physical boundaries define and protect your body, your personal space, and your sense of privacy. Other physical boundaries involve clothes, shelter, safety, money, space, noise, and so on.

Your physical boundaries need to be strong to protect you from harm. If you have a deep wound and it goes untreated you expose yourself to infection which can result in serious, life-threatening consequences. Protecting your physical boundaries is essential for your health and well-being.

Psychological Boundaries

Just as physical boundaries define who can touch us, how someone can touch us, and how close another may approach us, psychological boundaries define where our feelings end and another's begins. Many of us with eating challenges have a difficult time making this differentiation.

Psychological boundaries comprise the thinking part of who we are—what we put into our heads and what goes on inside there. This part of us is what we carry in our minds: our knowledge, wisdom, experience, memories, reflections, speculations, vocabulary, opinions, and, in some cases, the lies we've believed. It includes our emotions and thoughts, our will, intellect, mind, worldview, and pattern of thinking.

Psychological boundaries are important. They protect our sense of self-esteem and our ability to separate our feelings from the feelings of others. For example, do we take responsibility for our feelings and needs and allow others to do the same? Or do we feel overly responsible for other people's feelings and needs and neglect our own? Are we able to say no? Can we ask for what we need? Are we compulsive people-pleasers? Do we become upset simply because others around us are upset? Do we mimic the opinions of the people around us? The answers to these questions help us assess the strength of our psychological boundaries.

Having weak emotional boundaries is like getting caught in a hurricane with no protection. We are subject to and controlled by other people's feelings, and we can end up feeling bruised and battered.

This is also the area where we have responsibility to control our own bodies, where our own internal boundary conflicts reside. Self boundaries and false boundaries present themselves in this area.

Spiritual Boundaries

How can we set healthy boundaries, replace destructive habits, and undo the damage we've done to our bodies? How can our lives be characterized by such authentic signs as compassion, mercy, justice, and love, while at the same time maintaining healthy boundaries and a balanced life?

Quite simply, we cannot do this on our own. Our sinful nature will keep us from making the transformational changes we need to make. Only through God's help can we receive a new nature. Only by reorganizing our relationships and putting God first, understanding our responsibilities in Christ, and developing spiritual discipline can our lives begin to grow in the character of Christ.

Constructing a boundary of safety around our relationship with God is healthy. Within this boundary is a place where we make spiritual discipline a priority, including daily time with the Lord, reading the Word, praying, praising, worshipping, and developing our character to align with that of Christ.

Author June Hunt says,

> Long ago, I learned that we need to line up our thinking with God's thinking because a changed mind produces a changed heart, and a changed heart produces a changed life. That's the ultimate end: that we all experience a changed life through Christ and become all he created us to be.[3]

Boundaries Can Be Too Rigid or Too Loose

Those whose boundaries are too rigid shut everyone out of their lives. They appear aloof and distant and won't talk about feelings or show emotions. They exhibit extreme self-sufficiency and won't ask for help when they honestly need it. They won't allow anyone to get physically or emotionally close. They might as well live in a house surrounded by an immense wall with no gates. No one is allowed in.

On the other hand, those whose boundaries are too loose put their hands on strangers and let others touch them inappropriately. They may be sexually promiscuous, confuse sex with love, be driven to be in a sexual relationship, and get too close to others too fast. They may take on other people's feelings as their own, easily become emotionally overwhelmed, give too much, take too much, and be in constant need of reassurance. They may expect others to read their minds, think they can read other people's minds, say yes when they want to say no, and feel responsible for other people's feelings. Those with loose boundaries often lead chaotic lives, full of drama, as if they lived in houses with no locks, or even doors.

Violated Boundaries

All relationships should have limits on what is appropriate. Whether a boss is demanding more of you than should be expected or you are feeling victimized in your own marriage, a boundary violation is a serious matter. Many adult children of abuse (including verbal, physical, emotional, and sexual abuse) have no concept of how to set boundaries. They know walls, cell bars, and hiding places, but not boundaries. One of the after-effects of child abuse is the inability to either construct or enforce personal boundaries. However, this after-effect holds true no matter what our age:

When someone violates our boundaries it can be devastatingly hard for us to set healthy boundaries as life goes on.

Do you know when someone is violating your space—your personal boundary?

We begin our journey to freedom when we can be strong enough to let someone know they are overstepping our boundaries, either with our words or our actions. When we can say; "If you violate my territory (physically, verbally, emotionally, or mentally) then I will…" or, "This is my territory and you may not enter without my permission."

The Weight of Boundaries

The obesity epidemic comprises an estimated 72 million people in America—roughly 34 percent of our population. This figure doesn't take into consideration those who qualify as overweight, which is different from being obese.

Anne Katherine is a psychotherapist, licensed mental health counselor, and popular author who is known for her pioneering work in developing effective programs for recovery from food addiction and discovery of life's purpose. In her book *Boundaries: Where You End and I Begin,* she includes a special letter to overeaters that I found particularly powerful.

> If you are carrying extra weight, it may be providing you with a boundary as well.
>
> Weight is a good way to keep people at a distance when people have taken too much from you. It literally extends your physical boundary.
>
> If you were abused as a child, fat can feel like a comforting shield. It is a physical barricade against people who might harm you.
>
> Food and fat seem to protect us. Perhaps you eat more when you feel threatened. Perhaps you eat when you know someone is going to take more from you than you want to give. Perhaps you eat when you're with a person who assaults your boundaries.
>
> Boundary development is an important companion to an eating recovery program. Not until you know you can protect

yourself from intrusion and theft will you be safe without the extra weight.[4]

How Do We Know?

Do you wonder how to know if a lack of healthy boundaries is part of your life? If you can answer yes to one or more of the questions below, it may be time for you to start making different choices based on new personal property lines—that is, boundaries.

- Do some people take advantage of you?
- Do you sometimes have trouble saying no?
- Do you often suffer from feelings of guilt?
- Do you ever feel as though you have no control over some areas of your life?
- Do you try to have too much control over some areas of your life?
- Do you avoid conversations you know you should have?
- Do you wish you could be more assertive and in control?
- Do you lose patience with certain people or personality types?
- Do you feel anxious before a difficult conversation?
- Do you think of what you "should have" said after the conversation is over?
- Do you know when someone is violating your space?

God calls us to be good stewards of *everything* He has given to us and *every* blessing He bestows, but often we interpret that to mean the tangible external blessings He has provided—like family, friends, employment, finances, and worldly goods. But long before those external blessings He gave us something far greater. First, He gave us the physical vehicle—the vessel—to carry out His purpose and plan for our lives, followed by the glorious gift of His plans!

For you created my inmost being;

you knit me together in my mother's womb.
I praise you because I am fearfully and wonderfully made;
your works are wonderful,
I know that full well.
My frame was not hidden from you
when I was made in the secret place,
when I was woven together in the depths of the earth.
Your eyes saw my unformed body;
all the days ordained for me were written in your book
before one of them came to be (Psalm 139:13-16 NIV).

"For I know the plans I have for you," declares the LORD,
"plans to prosper you and not to harm you, plans to give you
hope and a future" (Jeremiah 29:11 NIV).

Now That We Understand Boundary Basics

The journey to find sanity doesn't happen overnight. It isn't just a matter of understanding what the word means or what types of boundaries exist, although these are important things to know. Understanding boundaries really begins when we stop seeing ourselves as helpless and drowning and realize how much power we have over our actions and emotions. More importantly, understanding boundaries is also becoming aware of what God's Word teaches us about the critical aspect of protecting our hearts. One of the most powerful actions we can take in life is to choose to be in relationships that bring out the best in us, that nurture our heart, and that allow us to bring out the best in others as well.

We must ask ourselves, "Am I treating the vessel God has given me with honor, respect, and love? Is the person I am today the person God is calling me to be? Is my relationship with food and eating bringing out the best in me? If God has made a difference in my life, am I a walking, talking, visual example of that difference?"

Chapter 4

It's All About Balance

I grew up going to the Ringling Brothers and Barnum & Bailey Circus every year as a child. The tightrope walking acts both fascinated and terrified me. Every step taken was intentional—deliberate—and firmly grasping the balancing pole was instrumental to get the performer safely from one side to the other.

Let's think of God as our balancing pole. We are walking on a tightrope every day of our life. When we firmly grasp God's principles, plans, and purpose for our lives, we can securely put one foot in front of the other and make it safely to the other side of any trial, tribulation, or turmoil. But our steps need to be intentional and deliberate choices—choices based on balancing our relationships, responsibilities, and boundaries.

In an interview with Crystal G. Martin, journalist and *Today Show* anchor Ann Curry shared her perspective on life after a health scare precipitated a conversation with her physician. The doctor warned her that unless she made significant changes in her life she was at risk for serious consequences. "In the time since I had that chat with my doctor, I've learned to be deliberate about how I spend my time on this Earth. I choose to fill my days with what I'm passionate about, and live with purpose. In the end, I want to be able to say, 'My life was what I made it.'"[1]

As Christians, let's take that one step further. Yes, our lives are what we make them, but combined with God's love, grace, and mercy, they can be so much more!

Intentional and Deliberate

We're told that the key to happiness and health is to "live a balanced life," but what does that really mean? What exactly are we supposed to balance? I used to think this phrase referred primarily to our working and playing, to the amount of time we spent in labor versus leisure. However, I've come to learn it's much more.

My good friend Dr. Debra Peppers is an international speaker and the host of her own television talk show, *Shakin' the Salt with Dr. Peppers*. She is also the author of *It's Your Turn Now,* a powerful book about her 100-pound weight loss and amazing journey from being a high school dropout to being named Teacher of the Year.

Debra believes, as I do, that we need to find balance in life before we can successfully embark on any nutritional journey or achieve long-term weight loss. But like me, there was a time in her life when she was unsure what that meant, causing her to dig deeper until she came across a description of the six primary components that make up a life. Being the teacher that she is, Debra developed a helpful visual aid she uses in her book and also in many of the motivational talks she gives around the world.

This simple but enlightening diagram includes six pie-shaped slices that clearly identify the areas of life we need to balance. I call it the "Slice-of-Life Balance Pie." Debra has graciously allowed me to share her diagram, as well as an insight and exercises from her book.

> I use this diagram in my seminars to help us take a realistic look at how we need to keep our lives balanced. Notice the size of each piece of the pie and examine the categories closely. If there are only two key ideas and goals that I want you to get out of this entire chapter, they are *balance* and *inner peace!* No matter how distorted your own balance wheel might be, and no matter how little inner peace you have had in the past, you can change!
>
> Look closely at the diagram. Take a minute to make an honest estimation of the proportions you would give each of these six areas in your own life. You may have even left out one or two of the pieces—don't be alarmed. I was defunct in all of them! [2]

SLICE-OF-LIFE BLANCE PIE

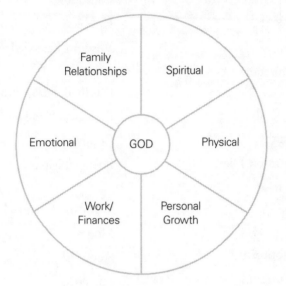

Before meeting Debra and reading her book, I had never seen a diagram like this. I had never learned the value of addressing all the areas of who I was. In my study, I had to admit that I, too, was defunct in many of them.

I've shared this diagram in my own workshops over the years, and you'd be surprised how many people have never understood the concept of what comprises a truly balanced life.

It's not that we're imbecilic nincompoops, we've just been busy with other things—like supporting families, making ends meet, juggling crisis and chaos, and dealing with issues as they arise. And unless we've been in some type of counseling or therapy, or the Holy Spirit has convicted us of this issue of balance in our lives, chances are we haven't spent a great deal of introspective time assessing the components that make up a balanced life.

Let's look briefly at each Slice-of-Life in Debra's Balance Pie to get a feel for what each area is *supposed* to contain.

Spiritual

Christian Growth

Bible Study

Prayer

Inspiration

Physical

Health

Nutrition/Diet

Exercise

Hygiene

Emotional

Heart/Soul

Mind/Feelings

Insight

Personal Growth

Education

Hobbies

Wisdom/Knowledge

Family Relationships

Biological Family

Family of God

Friends/Neighbors

Work and Financial

Money

Stewardship

Career/Job

When we are caught up in competition or even the everyday "rat-race" of life, it is hard to step back and take an honest assessment of what matters most in our life. We can be so busy and so intent on being "the winner" or being "the best" or "the richest" or "the thinnest" or "the most popular," that we forget what is really important in our lives—our faith, our family, our friends, forgiveness, and fun![3]

While it's good to be aware that our lives may need a bit of realignment to acquire healthy balance, it's also important to put this self-study introspection in proper perspective. I couldn't agree more with Oswald Chambers' insight:

We are not intended to understand Life. Life makes us what we are, but Life belongs to God. If I can understand a thing and can define it, I am its master. I cannot understand or define Life; I cannot understand or define God; consequently I am master of neither.[4]

Take a minute to make an honest estimation of the proportions you currently give each of these six areas in your own life—how much time you allocate to each section of your own Balance Pie. Now, grab your notebook and list each area on its own page, answering the following questions for each "slice of life."

1. Why have you allotted so much or so little time/resources to this area?

2. Do you *want* to give more time and focus to this area, even if you don't see how?

3. Do you feel you *should* give more time to this area, even if you don't really want to?

Praying for Insight

It's true, our lives belong to God, and as such we have a responsibility to Him. Although it is our responsibility to nurture our relationship with the Lord, it's also an honor, privilege, and blessing to be able to do so, especially through prayer.

> The Lord has ordained for you and me to pray His will into this world, into our own lives, and into the lives of family members. Prayer has always been the channel through which we come to know God by communicating with Him, as well as obtain His help in times of need, connect His super to our natural, and establish His dominion in our lives, our families, and in the world. From the beginning of time, God has intended for prayer to be His means of moving His promises out of the pages of the Bible and into the realities of our lives! Prayer is something God designed for us to use in order to possess His promises.[5]

A Word About the Work Slice-of-Life

In his book *How to Conquer Giants*, Duke Duvall shares an important aspect about one of the areas in our Balance Pie that is often unbalanced to the extreme: the area of work.

> Simply put, God blesses us when we work hard, when we diligently perform the tasks we set out to do. This is how we earn earthly wealth honestly. If we desire to achieve great things in this world, if we want to earn monetary riches, then we'll need to work hard in whatever field we have chosen.
>
> There is, however, a balance we must strike in this area of our lives if we are to be successful in the true and lasting sense. And in striking that balance, we must battle and defeat our next giant, the giant named Diversion. This giant wants us to make our work the very center of our lives, to the very point where we discount all other things including our families, our friends, our health, and even our God...Without a doubt, this is not the way God intended it to be.[6]

Indeed, it is not. Some of us may struggle with the emotional side effects of not setting the appropriate boundaries at the appropriate time. Just because we have felt unable in the past to make healthy choices in circumstances or relationships doesn't mean we're doomed to continue the same course. We can jump off the gerbil wheel of insanity at any time—and into the arms of a loving Father who will never forsake us.

Chapter 5

Basic Biology and Destructive Dieting

Not all diets are destructive. What is destructive, however, is what we're doing to our bodies when we frequently start and stop weight-loss programs.

In a recent healthy eating article in *MORE* magazine, Peter Jaret wrote about how weight-loss efforts are statistically futile—and how you can boost your health big time without dropping a pound.

> Dropping pounds through dieting has been shown to cause some health problems, including reduced bone mass, which increases the risk for osteoporosis. But the biggest problems probably result from weight cycling, or yo-yo dieting, which is the reality for most people who try to lose weight. Weight cycling has been linked to a host of concerns, including raised cholesterol levels, higher blood pressure, increased inflammation, insulin resistance and even depressed immune function. Consider high blood pressure, which is often associated with obesity. When researchers at the German Institute of Human Nutrition in Potdam-Rehbrucke looked at more than 12,000 middle-aged men and women for a study published in 2005, they found that obese men and women whose weight fluctuated over a two-year period were four times as likely to develop hypertension as the obese people whose weight remained stable. An earlier Italian study reported that women who had lost weight at least five times in five years were more likely to have high blood pressure than those whose weight remained stable.[1]

What is this telling us? Diets don't work and at some point can become harmful.

We're learning to set healthy boundaries with our adult children and the difficult people who push our buttons and make life challenging. Yet we can't seem to get a handle on this issue of food—and weight. We're growing older and wiser…but not thinner.

Scientists, researchers, and medical professionals have conducted countless studies over the years on weight loss, self-control, exercise, food cravings and addictions, and, of course, on dieting. The authors of *Change Anything* highlight one such study from the Stanford University medical school.

> Before we get too depressed, let's travel to Stanford University's medical school, where scholars examined the commercial diets people most often use for weight loss…These researchers found that every one of the most popular diets "worked." It turns out things aren't so bad after all. We now have carefully crafted plans to help us counteract our inborn cravings.
>
> And now for the not-so-good news—the news you already know—the diets worked only for people who stuck with them, and pretty much nobody did. Bummer.
>
> So the secret to wellness isn't in the diet or exercise program itself. Any approach that causes you to eat less and exercise more will lead to weight loss and improved fitness. Balanced diets and well-crafted exercise plans—along with shortcuts, secret ingredients, and fat-burning gizmos—all work (and work only) if they result in fewer calories ingested and more calories burned. And they work only if you keep them up—because tomorrow you will be eating again. Several times.[2]

That said, whether or not you have good self-control, or whether or not you exercise, if you go on a diet the odds are that you won't permanently lose weight, as the authors of *Willpower* corroborate.

> One reason is basic biology. When you use self-control to go through your in-box or write a report or go jogging, your body doesn't react viscerally. It's not physically threatened by your

decision to pay bills instead of watch television. It doesn't care whether you're writing a report or surfing the Web. The body might send you pain signals when you exercise too strenuously, but it doesn't treat jogging as an existential threat. Dieting is different. As the young Oprah Winfrey discovered, the body will go along with a diet once or twice—but then it starts fighting back. When fat lab rats are put on a controlled diet for the first time, they'll lose weight. But if they're then allowed to eat freely again, they'll gradually fatten up, and if they're put on another diet it will take them longer to lose the weight this time. Then, when they once again go off the diet, they'll regain the weight more quickly than the last time. By the third or fourth time they go through this boom-and-bust cycle, the dieting ceases to work; the extra weight stays on even though they're consuming fewer calories.[3]

Oh my.

It's too bad we didn't grasp this basic biology wisdom several decades ago before we got caught up in the yo-yo dieting, weight cycling, and boom-and-bust cycles.

But it is what it is, so what can we do now?

For starters, I'm going to advocate the three rules presented in *Willpower*:

1. Never go on a diet.

2. Never vow to give up chocolate or any other food.

3. Whether you're judging yourself or judging others, never equate being overweight with having weak willpower.[4]

Behind the Scenes

When it comes to the physical mechanics of the bodies God has provided to His children, I can understand being overwhelmed by it all, the technical information on how our bodies work, the chemical basis for our need to eat, how the body stores fat and uses sugar, and the physical consequences of overeating and destructive dieting. It's all quite involved and quite miraculous!

After all, we're talking about things like:

endorphins	dynorphins
tryptophan	enkephalins
serotonin	blood-brain barrier
amino acids	protein
insulin	stress triggers
blood sugar levels	metabolically caused cravings

In her book *Anatomy of a Food Addiction*, Anne Katherine has written one of the best resources I've ever read (that I could actually understand) on the brain chemistry of overeating. She opened my eyes to what's really going on internally when high-fat, high-sugar, and high-carb foods go into our mouths. After thoroughly explaining the chemical basis for why we overeat, she effectively sums up the chapter by explaining that many of us struggling with weight loss and yo-yo dieting were born "sensitive to pain." Her perspective gave me valuable insight in a way other diet book explanations did not.

Because of insufficient serotonin levels, when you are hurt, you really hurt. If your parents were not skilled at parenting, if they made mistakes with you, it hurt bad.

Sugar and other carbohydrates brought you relief. Carbohydrates affected your endorphin functioning and caused tryptophan to enter your brain cells. Tryptophan manufactured serotonin and it was released. This made you less sensitive to pain, lowered your anxiety, helped you relax, and made you less aware. The increased endorphins stopped emotional and physical pain and gave you pleasure...These various endorphins made you crave more sugar, starch, and/or fat...

Human beings learn pain relief very quickly. If something works to stop our pain, we try it again...If crying brings Mom with warmth and reassurance, we cry again. If eating sugar brings relief and the end of pain, we will eat sugar again.

We ate sugar again. Again it caused the release of

endorphins and serotonin. Sugar brought us relief from pain...We ate more sugar. The more we ate, the better we felt. We did not know we were changing the endorphin receptors in our brains...But we may have noticed, as we grew older, that we could eat more sugar than our friends. They would be satisfied with one piece. We weren't satisfied with a bagful.[5]

For many of us, overwhelming physical cravings for sugar, starch, and fat dominate our lives. Some days it's a creamy milkshake or ice cream, a hamburger with French fries, or maybe potato chips and dip. Other days it's mouthwatering flaky pastry or freshly baked bread with real butter and jam. These physical cravings have a basis in chemistry.

Address the Stress

Stress-hunger is a compelling, sometimes overwhelming hunger based not on the body's need for food but on erroneous hormonal messages. Studies have also proven that the greater the number of failed diets you've been on, the greater the likelihood that stress-eating has been your downfall. Now let's say we combine all of that with the added fact that as a society we have an incredibly difficult time setting boundaries, and we have a recipe for disaster.

Here's another helpful explanation for what's going on physically when stress increases:

> In just the last few years, landmark scientific studies into the causes of stress-eating have revealed the power of two stress hormones, cortisol and its sidekick adrenaline, to summon four other hormones.
>
> These four hormones, aptly termed the Masters of Metabolism, include ghreline (the hunger hormone), serotonin (the satisfaction hormone), oxytocin (the hormone of affection, bonding, and sexuality), and leptin (the weight-loss regulator). These Masters of Metabolism, in combination with insulin, cortisol, and adrenaline, dictate how strongly you will crave food, how much you'll want to eat, how much weight you'll put on, and in what area of your body the fat will be deposited.

These hormones respond to your thoughts, feelings, and the world around you. In an attempt to help you deal with the stresses of daily life, they can send you virtually undeniable commands to seek out food and, after making it taste extraordinarily good, command your body to store that food energy away as fat.

Sheer willpower can hold these hormones at bay for only so long. Even as you deny yourself the food they make you crave, they will become more efficient at turning food energy into fat. So, even if you eat no more than you have in the past—or even less—you'll still gain weight. To make matters worse, they'll probably direct your body to store it around your middle.[6]

If you're prone to stress-eating, you probably know of certain situations that trigger you to overeat. Some common triggers are:

- Skipping breakfast
- Repeated dieting
- Diet drinks
- Lack of sleep
- Overweight friends
- Certain types of viruses
- Aggravating friends or family
- Sitting at a computer or desk for most of the day

A Deadly Duo

If you've ever observed a recovering alcoholic or drug addict, you know that he must work vigorously to maintain his sobriety, even years afterwards. Anne Katherine explains why.

He's over the worst of alcohol withdrawal in a week (unless he's also used other drugs), he's in better physical shape after a few months, and his body has repaired most of the damage after a couple of years. So why must he keep going to A.A. meetings? Why are sober alcoholics still attending meetings 20 years later? Because anyone who uses a substance to cope with life has learned two deadly principles: avoidance and substitution.

Alcohol, drugs, sugar, and eating are all effective ways to avoid living and feeling. Once we've learned avoidance, we can automatically slip into it again. The next new stress can trigger us into avoidance without our spotting it.

We have also learned substitution. We've learned to substitute a substance for a real need. Anytime we eat because we're lonely, we are substituting food for the answer to our loneliness. Food doesn't actually fix the loneliness. It's still there, but food is used as a substitute for a friend. When we eat because we're afraid, we are substituting food for what would help us to be less afraid. When we eat because we worked too hard, we are substituting food for not taking care of ourselves.

Once we've learned to substitute something for a real need, we can confuse ourselves. You're thirsty, you eat. You're tired, you eat. The appropriate response to thirst is to drink; to tiredness, to rest. Food is the wrong answer and eventually we get confused and lose track of the real problem.[7]

What Is the Real Problem?

What do you think we really hunger for? What is it you hunger for late at night, after everyone's gone to bed and it's just you and your emotions and the food calling your name? The anonymous author of *Listen to the Hunger* has an idea.

We hunger for security, for accomplishment, for love, for adventure, for spiritual growth. Our hunger reflects and expresses our needs, and our needs pyramid one on top of the other. We satisfy one hunger, and we move on to the next, and we go back to the beginning and do it again.

Do you think underneath all the striving, the wanting, the doing, and the moving, we each have a deep, basic hunger for peace? Is that what some of the eating is about? How effective

a tranquilizer is food? Isn't there a better way to settle our rest-
lessness and our anxiety?

Food is a temporary tranquilizer. We can eat ourselves into
a kind of oblivion where we no longer feel or care.[8]

Pounds of Pain and Protection

During my pregnancy at the age of 16, I began to stuff down an
increasingly painful emptiness and hopelessness with food. I ate to avoid
feeling. Food was most definitely my tranquilizer when I was afraid—and
I was afraid a lot. Gaining 100 pounds with my pregnancy was the start
of a battle with weight and dieting that would last for more than 30 years.
After my son's birth and before I became a Christian, I added recreational
drugs, alcohol, and empty relationships to the mix.

A pattern developed over the years with regards to my weight. Using
various extreme deprivation diets, including diet pills, shots, and liquid
protein fasts, I would drop significant amounts of weight in short periods of time. Over the years my weight would drastically fluctuate from
150 to 190 to 230 to 130 to 180 to 200 to 175—up and down and up and
down. My highest recorded weight was 280 pounds the day I had my
weight loss surgery, but I know there was a time when I was dangerously
close to 300 pounds.

I didn't understand the basic biology of body chemistry, or what I was
doing to my body every time I stressfully starved myself into submission
on another diet.

During those years it never occurred to me I was fighting a useless battle with equally useless tools. My paternal grandmother and my mother
both struggled with obesity, yet I blamed only myself for having poor willpower, for being weak and pitiful—never thinking about the fact I had
grown up modeling the behaviors of two emotionally repressed women
who had mastered the art of avoidance and substitution regarding their
own issues with food.

Back then no one ever talked about being overweight as a disease, a
generational curse, or a visible representation of an inability to set healthy
boundaries. Back then I didn't understand that everyone is born with
three inner needs—the needs for love, significance, and security. Back
then I didn't know what it was like to have any of those needs met.

As infants, we need someone to feed us, bathe us, dress us, change our diapers, and keep us warm and safe. We need to be held, protected, and loved. We are entirely dependent. Although our dependency level may change as we mature, our needs do not.

In my life, love, significance, and security were largely unmet needs, leaving me with an aching emptiness. For many years the only way I could keep the pain manageable was to dull it with drugs, empty relationships, and food. When I became a Christian at 35, drugs were the first to go, followed by the empty relationships, leaving me the one thing I could depend on to help me avoid the truth—the one tranquilizer guaranteed to dull my pain. Food.

Destructive Dieting

I'm not going to spend a lot of time sharing my destructive diet history in these pages because it would easily require an entire chapter. Suffice it to say that chances are you and I could share a lot of the same diet horror stories, such as what happens to the inside of your mouth when you eat pineapple for weeks, or how your digestive tract fares when it processes nothing but vegetables for a month, or how sore your arms get from daily HCG shots, or how humiliating it is to get on that scale in front of a group of people to discover that you gained 10 pounds since you were last there.

Enough is enough.

This next writing exercise is going to prove to be quite the trip down memory lane for most of us. Grab your journal and at the top of a new page write this heading: *Every Diet I Can Remember*. Now, start writing down every diet you've ever been on. It isn't important to get them in any kind of chronological order, and I can guarantee that the more you really think about it you're going to find yourself remembering diets that you have long forgotten. Write about the results you had on the diets, how long they lasted, how you felt when you were on them…anything you can remember.

Completing this exercise will provide empowering truth as you move forward on this new journey toward setting boundaries and finding sanity.

Chapter 6

Our Mighty Memories of Food

Our bond with food is strong, and when we use it as a substance to avoid or substitute a feeling, we can find ourselves thinking about eating day and night, as Anne Katherine describes:

> Whenever I went anywhere or did anything, the food was the major attraction. I went to the fair to eat the special foods that only fairs have. I went to the movies to eat popcorn. I went out with friends in order to have dinner or lunch. If there had been such a thing as a party without food, I probably wouldn't have gone.[1]

Until prompted to write them down, I never realized that some of my most vivid memories from my childhood included food. When it comes to understanding the role food plays in our lives, it's important to understand how our relationship with it developed in the first place. How we see food—and remember food—and what place it holds in the memories of our hearts.

Grab your notebook and start a new page with this heading, *My Mighty Memories of Food*. Then, answer the following questions. Include as much detail as possible, especially if you can remember how you felt during those times.

1. What are your first recollections of food and eating?

2. Are there specific foods that trigger memories for you— positive or negative?

3. What were mealtimes like for you growing up? What are they like now?

Some of my earliest memories of food reflect the financial struggles my mom experienced in order to provide it.

Growing up in a single-parent household, the years we spent as welfare recipients are forever imprinted on my memory. Living first in the projects on Cleveland's east side, and then in the downstairs unit of a west side rental house, we were fortunate to have a roof over our heads, and it wasn't until I was an adult that I fully understood how poor we really were.

Mom struggled to make ends meet and frequent trips to the welfare office were commonplace for us. We spent hours standing in line for food stamps. Much of the food we received monthly was stamped with the same big block letters and although it's been decades, I can still see the acronym AFDC in my mind's eye—Aid for Dependent Children. It was a long time before I realized that some people—most people—grew up with *liquid* milk, not the AFDC powder that Mom carefully mixed with water.

We lived on high-carbohydrate staples like goulash, macaroni and cheese, potatoes, rice, and cereal. Fancy meat like ham and turkey only came by way of well-dressed strangers who would stop by around Thanksgiving or Christmas with boxes of food and canned goods and whose visits always made my mom cry.

Mealtimes were hard for Mom. There's a certain amount of synchronicity that goes into preparing, cooking, and serving several dishes at one time. Mom couldn't quite master that skill, but God bless her, she tried. We ate primarily at the small Formica kitchen table or on folding metal TV trays in the living room watching programs like *Lassie, Lost in Space, I Dream of Jeannie,* or *I Love Lucy*. On Sunday, we loved to follow Mitch Miller's bouncing ball during his weekly sing-along program and then watch *The Wide World of Disney.*

Dinnertime in my family didn't resemble the Cleaver household of *Leave It to Beaver*. Plus, Mom worked a lot of odd jobs for Manpower Temporary and there were many times she wasn't home to fix dinner. We'd have to fend for ourselves with help from our older sister, when her nose wasn't buried in a book. If it was, my brother, Greg, and I were only too happy to see what culinary concoction we could dream up. (Roasting marshmallows over the flames of the gas stovetop burner comes to mind.)

Never Underestimate the Power of the Pen

You may recall earlier when I shared how integral journaling has been in my own healing and personal growth. This is a good example because my decades-old notes show that this particular food memory exercise jarred loose another memory that held significance in my life, helping me to connect more of the puzzle pieces to eventually reveal the entire picture, including lost pieces that, once retrieved, made the picture so much clearer.

No matter how hard I tried to avoid it, I spilled something at the dinner table on a pretty regular basis. It's not that I was a hyperactive child. The spill was usually the result of being startled by a sudden shout or movement, as I was easily frightened. I was afraid a great deal of the time as a young girl.

Mealtime memories can play a significant role in understanding who we are and why we respond as we do to food. They can also help us unlock painful memories, enabling us to move forward in areas in our lives that have held us in bondage.

In a questionnaire I distributed as part of my research for this book, Phyllis wrote about her early mealtime memories. "In my home, dinnertime was a solemn and silent experience. Our father believed the axioms 'Silence is golden' and 'Don't speak unless you're spoken to,' and he seldom spoke to us, or to our mother, for that matter. The only happy memories I have around eating were the times Grandma would visit and she would make my dad's favorite dessert, the richest black forest cake you've ever tasted. She was from Germany and this was a recipe that she was famous for in the town where she lived. Those times Dad smiled and laughed and it was like he was a different person."

It wasn't until years later, when Phyllis tipped the scales at over 300 pounds, that she came to understand how she was meeting her unmet needs as an adult by recreating the only times she felt happy and loved as a child—the times when she could eat the richest desserts possible.

Buying Our Own Food

I distinctly remember the first time I bought food in a grocery store on my own, with my own money, without my mother. Not at Pell's Deli across the street from our house, but at the A&P Grocery Store on Lorrain Avenue, a good mile or two from home.

I got the money from redeeming glass soda pop bottles. Back then, there were no recycling centers or organized programs and you could redeem collected bottles at most neighborhood delicatessens or grocery stores. Because this provided a source of instant cash, as kids we kept our eyes open for these valuable commodities, which were mostly Coca-Cola, Dr Pepper, Pepsi, and the emerald green 7-Up bottles.

After a particularly fruitful pop bottle scavenge, my brother, Greg, and I had some money of our own and we were going to spend it. Product advertising had done its job and there was a new food creation on everyone's tongue (both literally and figuratively). We were determined to try it. The adventure was all very secretive and quite grown-up. I was about twelve and Greg was nine. We didn't have bikes and although I don't recall the walk *to* the store, I vividly recall the walk—the run—back home.

Our one purchase that day?

A tub of Cool Whip.

It was the first time in history a whipped cream-like product could be distributed in a frozen state and kept in the refrigerator. It represented a major breakthrough in food preservation. But that aspect didn't matter to us as we had no intention of preserving it. Our goal was to eat it—all of it—before we returned home, thereby eliminating any evidence of our unapproved grocery store journey.

We didn't plan on the product being a solid chunk of frozen cream, but that didn't stop us from using our fingers to scoop it out, passing the white plastic tub back and forth until it was empty. We practically inhaled the sweet concoction and quickly disposed of the container in an alley trash can. The roiling in my stomach began almost immediately. I fought the urge to get sick, running all the way home with my brother shouting, "Wait up! Wait up!"

I don't recall ever being so nauseated in my life. If my brother was in the same boat I've blocked it out, because once we got home all I can remember is sitting on the bathroom floor next to the toilet, trying (unsuccessfully) to keep my long hair out of the water as I leaned over the edge of the bowl for what seemed like hours.

To my knowledge Mom never discovered our secret escapade.

As uncomfortable as that experience was, it represented a significant milestone in my life, a time when buying my own food made me feel powerful, in control, and safe. It also ushered in the start of a sugar addiction that would become my drug of choice for decades.

Can you recall buying your first food? If so, how did it make you feel? What memories do you have of shopping with your mother or father? Use your journal and write down any childhood memories you have of food. You might have to drill deep to recall memories, but they're a bit like cockroaches—once you let one in, a whole lot more will follow.

I have fond memories of shopping with our mom at the West Side Market where a gloriously abundant supply of fruits, vegetables, and meat was on display and where my relationship with penny candy was born and nurtured. This was also where I first saw how food looked "in the raw," where it really came from, when my brother and I would dart up and down the aisles peering into refrigerated glass display cases looking for things that would gross us out, like pig's feet, cow tongues, intestines, and various organ meats like brains and livers. One case even had horse heads (I never have figured out what people did with those—make soup, maybe?). Anything we could squeal over and gawk at was our goal—we were such typical city kids.

I also remember Mom taking us to buy freshly made perogies (a Polish stuffed dumpling) almost every week from women wearing babushkas in the basement of an ornate church in the flats of Cleveland. I wonder if Greg remembers it, but I would guess this is where my brother first connected with music, as he loved to sit at the old upright piano in the church basement, pounding on the keys as Mom stood in line. It seemed we were always standing in some type of food line.

I also vividly recall the times as a little girl when we were able to eat at the restaurant with the two huge golden arches stretching across the entire building, one on each side. You couldn't go inside; you could only use the drive-thru or park in the small adjacent lot and walk up to the window. We always parked in the lot and sometimes Mom let us walk up to the window with her, but most times we sat nearby at one of the concrete picnic tables as my older sister tried to keep my younger brother and me out of mischief. There was a sign outside that read "We have sold over 10,000," an astronomical number I couldn't begin to fathom.

Eating out was a rare treat reserved for very special occasions, and knowing the paper bag Mom carried back to the table always contained a perfectly wrapped hamburger for each of us was a really big deal. Sometimes, on extra special occasions, we got to share a bag of what I was certain had to be the world's best French fries.

Today, the outdoor signs that reach high into the air read, "Billions and Billions Served," and McDonald's is now the single largest purchaser of beef in the United States, at nearly a billion pounds a year. Today the golden arches I remember are long gone, yet this powerful memory lingers on—one that viscerally connects food with feelings of love, significance, and security—the three inner needs we are all born with, the three things I always seemed to be searching for but could seldom find. Three things I could depend on finding, the older I got, anytime I reached into a brown bag covered with advertising slogans and pulled out a perfectly wrapped burger made especially for me.

Do you have any fast-food memories? We're going to talk more about the implications of fast food later, as a means to instantly gratify unmet needs and quickly anesthetize emotions, but for now please start a new page in your journal and at the top of it write *Fast-Food Memories*. Then, write as much as you can remember.

Making Sense of Memories

For the most part, the majority of my childhood memories involving food are quite pleasant—one of the reasons it has been a powerful substitute to help me avoid facing the truth of painful emotions or situations in adulthood. It makes sense that we wouldn't use something that called to mind negative feelings when we're trying to avoid negative feelings by stuffing them down with food.

Some people have only negative memories of eating and food as they were growing up, especially those suffering from anorexia and bulimia. However, for the most part those of us who are compulsive emotional eaters or yo-yo dieters, many of our childhood food memories bring warmth, comfort, and feelings of protection and love.

But no matter how you slice it, serve it, or eat it, *food is not love.*

Chapter 7

God Is Love—Food Is Not

At the beginning of our lives we were helpless. Someone took care of us and fed us, or we wouldn't be here today. As we got older, we could feed ourselves if someone gave us food and utensils. During our school years, we ate in the school cafeteria or brought a lunchbox. At home, we learned to eat what was provided or prepare and consume meals and snacks on our own. By the time we were living on our own or married, most of us were capable of taking care of our nutritional needs, either through buying and preparing food, eating out, or a combination of both. The anonymous author of *Listen to the Hunger* writes about this connection:

> If we were lucky, there was warmth, tenderness, approval, and fun, as well as calories. Most likely from time to time, there was some anger, hostility, and anxiety during meals. What was consistent, as long as one or more people were present with us while we were eating, was a sense of connectedness. Even if we ate with a caretaker who sat with us in stony silence, someone was there. We were not alone...
>
> The connection is still there. Food means, if not love, at least interrelatedness. For the time while I am eating, I am not alone in a cold, cruel world. There is the memory, conscious or unconsciousness, of someone nearby who is looking after me and my needs. I feel relatively secure, if only for the moment. And so, I like to eat. When did I start eating more for emotional comfort and support than for bodily need? Were the two ever separate? How did the emotional factor so eclipse

the physical one that I could overeat to the point of damaging my body?[1]

In my journey of piecing together the fragments of my life, I can clearly see when I started eating for emotional comfort, when I began to use food as a substitute for love. Can you? If so, take some time to write about it in your journal.

Author Geneen Roth wrote in her book *When Food Is Love: Exploring the Relationship Between Eating and Intimacy*, "I will never have a happy childhood. I missed it: the love, the acceptance, the feeling that I mattered. I missed it the first time around and I will never get that chance again. I have been railing against that for twenty years. But railing isn't healing. Healing is another story."[2] Pastor Tiz Huch corroborates Roth's emotions:

> It is sad but true that many men and women around the world suffer the long-term effects of never having received genuine love from one or both of their parents. These individuals may appear at ease on the outside, but on the inside they have deep voids longing to be filled. The results of hurt and rejection can be far-reaching, and a crushed spirit can lead to many destructive behavior patterns. As we said before, emotional problems that aren't dealt with don't go away; they go underground, only to resurface months or years later. That is why it is crucial to deal with any emotional issues and to break the ties that they hold on us as early as possible.[3]

It's important to express and receive love in a healthy way, and sometimes people who have used food to avoid heart issues find that hard to do.

Sadly, for many of us love looks a lot like an all-you-can-eat buffet. A place where we can help ourselves to as much "love" as our plates will hold and go back for more—and more. But in the end this one-sided love will never fill the emptiness, it will never provide the connectedness we need, and it will never, ever, care about our hearts, souls, and spirits.

The Heart of the Matter

The heart of the gospel message is gaining compassion for others—

trying to love the unlovable. But what if the unlovable ones are us? What if we have no compassion for ourselves—if all we have is self-loathing and hatred for what we have become? What if every gauge we use to measure our own self-worth is associated with our weight?

Alas, this isn't far off the mark when it comes to describing those of us who have used food as a false boundary, as a way to avoid or substitute our real feelings, real needs.

The Bible says that we were created in God's image—fearfully and wonderfully made. Perhaps the time has come to stop beating ourselves up and start viewing ourselves as precious and perfect children of God, no matter what we weigh. This doesn't mean we resign ourselves to being unhealthy, overweight, or obese. It doesn't mean we give up the goal to get in better shape. It means that right now, this very minute and for all eternity, God loves us and will always be here to guide us even when we don't understand His plan. This truth does not change whether we weigh 130, 230, or 330 pounds or more. God does not pour out or withhold His love based on how much we weigh.

> Setting boundaries with food begins with a change of heart—not with a change of digits on your bathroom scale.

Yes, life has dealt some of us a cruel and bitter hand. The trials and tribulation we've experienced have been considerable, and the seemingly never-ending succession of gut-wrenching blows to our hearts and spirits never seems to stop. But if you're reading this now, you are far from the point of no return. You are not a victim of situations or circumstances, and the choices you have made in the past need not sentence you to a life of bondage.

Leslie Vernick's insight gives us food for thought in *The Truth Principle* as she writes about this need for a deep-seated change of heart:

> How we act and live stems from what is in our heart. A change of heart requires much more than simply changing sinful behaviors into more Christ-like behaviors. A change of heart requires us to allow God to rearrange the desires of our heart. The things that motivate us in our natural self most should no longer control us; instead, the love of Christ should control us,

the glory of God should control us, and the mind of Christ should control us.[4]

In order to conquer the weight-weariness that pervades our soul, let's ask God to rearrange the desires of our heart. Let's ask Him to help us see ourselves through His eyes and understand how special we are to Him.

God Chose Us!

In 1 Peter 2:9, the Bible says that we are "God's very own possession." Max Lucado reminds us that we are a chosen people:

> Do you ever feel unnoticed? New clothes and styles may help for a while. But if you want permanent change, learn to see yourself as God sees you: "He has covered me with clothes of salvation and wrapped me with a coat of goodness, like a bridegroom dressed for his wedding, like a bride dressed in jewels" (Isaiah 61:10 NCV).
>
> Does your self-esteem ever sag? When it does, remember what you are worth. "You were bought, not with something that ruins like gold or silver, but with the precious blood of Christ, who was like a pure and perfect Lamb" (1 Peter 1:18-19 NCV).
>
> The challenge is to remember that. To meditate on it. To focus on it. To allow his love to change the way you look at you.[5]

Ahh...the way we look at ourselves—therein lays the challenge. In her book *Seeing Yourself Through God's Eyes*, June Hunt addresses this vital component.

> *Identity.* What would it be like to not know your own identity—to have *spiritual amnesia*? If you don't know who you are, you cannot experience deep inner peace and complete contentment—for instead, confusion reigns. Sadly, this is how many people live today—they simply don't know who they are. But you do not have to live this way. The key is to learn to *see yourself through God's eyes*.[6]

In his bestselling book *Experiencing God*, Henry Blackaby describes how God pursues a love relationship with us that leaves no doubt that fellowship with God the Father will change our lives.

> One of our church members always was having difficulty in his personal life, in his family, at work, and in the church. One day I went to him and asked, "Can you describe your relationship with God by sincerely saying, 'I love you with all my heart'?" The strangest look came over his face. He said, "Nobody has ever asked me that. No, I could not describe my relationship with God that way. I could say I obey him, I serve him, I worship him, and I fear him. But I cannot say that I love him."
>
> I realized that everything in his life was out of order because God's basic purpose for his life was out of order. God created us for a love relationship with Him. If you cannot describe your relationship with God by saying that you love Him with all your being, then you need to ask the Holy Spirit to bring you into that kind of a relationship.[7]

Hope Comes from the Heart

I've finally come to understand what trusting relationships look like as I've developed a relationship with a trustworthy God. In Paul's letter to the Philippians he said, "And this is my prayer: that your love may abound more and more in knowledge and depth of insight" (Philippians 1:9 NIV).

When our priority becomes the development of an intimate and loving relationship with Jesus, the sand in the hourglass of life shifts.

> Don't copy the behavior and customs of this world, but let God transform you into a new person by changing the way you think. Then you will learn to know God's will for you, which is good and pleasing and perfect (Romans 12:2).

In her book *The Truth Principle*, Leslie Vernick speaks of how loving God changes us from the inside out.

> The process of personal growth, Christian maturity, fruitfulness, and becoming more and more like Christ begins with seeds of love sown in our heart. Christ often used the

metaphor of garden life as a teaching tool. An apple tree cannot bear figs, can it? Why not? Because the very essence of the apple tree is defined by its roots, which are apple-tree roots and not fig-tree roots. Apples are a natural outgrowth of the roots. We will never have Christ likeness or the fruit of the spirit in our lives if our roots are shallow, underdeveloped, diseased, or of a different stock.

What are the roots of Christian living? The roots are love. Jesus tells us that we cannot bear fruit unless we are rooted in Him (John 15). Just as a branch is in essence and nature like the vine from which it sprouts, we are to reflect God's image in us. And God is love. He tells us that when we love Him we will obey Him. Rules don't bring heart obedience, but love does.[8]

God is love—not food.

This powerful truth may be hard to grasp, especially if we're holding on to old baggage that needs to be unpacked and discarded.

Chapter 8

Experiencing Emotions

I once read that every extra pound we carry on our body is equal to a pound of emotional pain we're carrying in our heart. When it comes to looking at the part our emotions play in the drama of our life when we have weak or nonexistent boundaries, it's important to understand that our emotions are not the problem; they are the indication of a problem.

I love what Donna Carter writes about our emotions in her book *10 Smart Things Women Can Do to Build a Better Life*:

> Our emotional world is one of the most difficult parts of our lives to manage. We think we're in complete control, but then something or someone pushes our buttons and our emotions go from 0 to 60 faster than a Porsche. Later, in the aftermath, we wonder, "What was that all about?"[1]

Indeed…what is it all about? For many of us, this is the million-dollar question.

When psychotherapist Dr. Doreen Virtue first began writing about the link between childhood abuse and compulsive overeating, the idea was met with resistance. Today, the idea doesn't seem so farfetched. Dr. Virtue found that when women turn to food for comfort, security, and sometimes self-punishment, in the majority of cases the overeating was brought on by emotionally painful and traumatic events including incest, rape, abuse, molestation, the death of a loved one, job problems, financial worries…the list goes on. She is quick to point out that not every person who is battling an eating problem has been sexually or physically abused.

Many women struggle with overeating that stems from stress, depression, anxiety, relationship problems, and career troubles. But no matter the core issue, she found that once the pain is released, the insatiable appetite for food is no longer present.

> Our appetite for food is usually an accurate reflection of whether we're on the right track or not. When we are living a false life, one that runs counter to our deep, inner vision, we crave food. Instead of healing our life, we mask our problems with the bandage known as food. We act like incarcerated prisoners who, in order to better deal with the miserable state of existence, turn to drugs to numb the reality of life.[2]

Both subtle and not-so-subtle forms of abuse can scar us for life. We can be injured physically, emotionally, sexually, and yes, even spiritually. In all instances, it's going to be important to get at the root of our issues with food in order to begin releasing the pain. That begins with an important first step, as author Geneen Roth discovered.

> The first step in healing is telling the truth. When you tell the truth, you acknowledge your losses. When you acknowledge your losses, you grieve about them. When you grieve about them, you let go of defining yourself by how much and how badly you've been abused. You begin living in the present instead of living in reaction to the past.
>
> As long as you eat compulsively, your life is about what you eat, how much you eat, how much you weigh, and what you will look like, be like, when you stop eating compulsively. Your pain seems to be about food, willpower, and looking a certain way. But your pain is not about what it seems to be about. And if you don't know what your pain is about, you can't release yourself from it.[3]

In *Listen to the Hunger*, the author writes, "One of the ways to try to fix emotional and spiritual emptiness is to translate it into physical hunger and attempt to fill the inner void with food. There is never enough food to do the job, because food won't fill emotional and spiritual emptiness."[4]

She's correct—it won't. I know it and deep down you know it too. It's impossible to tell you how many times I have shut off my feelings with food. But the good news is that we can learn to experience our emotions fully, without the anesthetic of food. But it's going to take a willingness to be emotionally authentic and spiritually disciplined.

Emotional Authenticity

I spent decades battling a weight problem that had its origins in a time when weight wasn't the problem. Dealing with the demons of my past was only possible because of the transformational power of Jesus, the grace of God, the wisdom of the Holy Spirit, and the help of gifted counselors. Today, I've got an entirely different perspective on this issue of setting boundaries with food—and it's brought me renewed freedom. My greatest prayer is that you will become emotionally, spiritually, and physically ready for a radical change in life as well.

By the time we're desperate for sanity, our life experiences have been stacked layer upon layer like an elaborate cake, held together by the glue of sugar-coated truth, and now time has sliced into our towering confection of life and it's beginning to topple over, revealing layer after layer of pain.

Emotional authenticity requires that we do some deep self-introspection, including addressing the significant life issues that in our hearts we know are at the core of our being—issues such as domestic violence, childhood abuse and/or molestation, alcoholism, divorce, unhappy marriages, drug/alcohol/sex addictions, depression, bipolar disorders, and everything in between.

The Mind-Body Connection

You may think your thoughts are just your thoughts, that they're inside your head and that's where they end. Alas, that isn't the case. As author Jillian Michaels puts it,

> The way you think, even in the deepest part of your subconscious, affects your behavior in ways you can't see. Your behavior in turn shapes your reality, again in ways you often aren't aware of. Being as simplistic as possible, you could say that positive thinking makes us act in positive ways, setting in motion a chain reaction that turns a situation's outcome our way.[5]

Conversely, negative feelings can make us act in negative ways, turning a situation's outcome in a direction that can create or continue destructive patterns that last for years. In *Listen to the Hunger* the author writes,

> Unfortunately, because of powerful feelings that were too much for us to cope with at the time, we may have learned to short-circuit emotional reactions into false hunger signals. Instead of allowing ourselves to feel loneliness or anger or embarrassment, we immediately translate the unpleasant feelings into hunger. In this way we mask our true emotions and hide them from everyone, including ourselves.[6]

The Danger of Ignoring Emotions

Masking emotions was the story of my life—my family's way of life.

To say I grew up in a severely emotionally repressed environment would be an understatement. We never talked about anything of a personal nature in my home, as though feelings simply didn't exist. Intimate mother and daughter communication was foreign to my mom. In fact, she never told me about the "facts of life." I learned about monthly cycles and puberty in health class at school.

It wasn't that Mom was cold or cruel—far from it. She was joyful, hopeful, and possessed an adventuresome spirit that opened a lot of doors for us as kids. She lived for us and wanted to give us every experience she never had as a child. It's just that expressing emotions, especially painful ones, was incredibly difficult for her.

My mother never met her father and had survived horrific physical abuse at the hands of her mother. She ran away from home at 15 and never looked back. We were, quite literally, her only family. Although she never talked about it, her divorce from my father was devastating. She never remarried.

My mom believed that if you ignored difficult situations or traumatic issues they would eventually go away and be forgotten. If you swept the dust of pain under the rug, or off the porch and into the bushes, it would inevitably disappear. Out of sight and out of mind. Everything was sunshine and lollipops—even when it wasn't.

In his novel *Prince of Tides*, Pat Conroy portrays this same mindset in a powerful way when he writes of the narrator's (Tom Wingo) struggle to overcome the psychological damage inflicted by his dysfunctional childhood in South Carolina. At the age of 13, three escaped convicts invaded Tom's home and raped him along with his mother and sister. His older brother killed two of the aggressors with a shotgun, while his mother stabbed the third with a kitchen knife. She then instructs the children to help her bury the bodies, clean the blood off the walls in the house, take showers, and get dressed all in time to prepare dinner for the father of the house when he arrives home later that evening. She admonishes the children over and over again as they rush to erase all clues of the horrible event, saying, "It didn't happen, not a word of this ever again. It did not happen, it never happened. You hear me? It never happened." They buried the bodies beneath the house and never spoke of it again.

But it did happen, forever changing the emotional makeup of everyone concerned. Pretending otherwise didn't erase the memory. The older brother died and the sister developed a severe split personality disorder. A suicide attempt finally brought the sister the psychological help she needed. The protagonist developed a deep fear of intimacy, which affected his marriage to the point of adultery and near divorce.

Perhaps the dynamics of that fictional family scenario are a bit dramatic. However, if we look at our own past, many of us who use food to avoid feeling our emotions can find a time when "out of sight and out of mind" was the mantra that addressed our painful truths.

Many of us have bodies buried under the house. And we've learned to ignore them by stuffing down the pain with food.

Where It Began

Growing up in our house, the elephant in the room—the body buried under our house—was my debilitating fear of the dark. This was never addressed, but it was something I carried into my adult years. My need to be where it was light required that compensation be made for car trips that kept us out after dark, such as traveling with a flashlight or driving with the obnoxious reading light turned on. Lights were always left on throughout the house and especially at night. And when my younger brother joked around as younger brothers are apt to do—running from a room, turning off the light, and closing the door on me—he had no idea my screams of terror were real, coming from a repressed memory that lived within me like a parasitic dragon, roaring to life whenever I was thrust into darkness.

Nightmares woke me up virtually every night screaming. Sometimes I would open my mouth to scream and nothing would come out, as if I had no voice. I hated going to bed at night. It was a horrific way to live, and it was how I lived year after year after year.

As a little girl, I loved attending Vacation Bible School during summer when the bus would come by our neighborhood and pick us up. This was my only exposure to God. We did not attend church on a regular basis, nor was ours a Christian home in the sense that God was an active part of our upbringing. But there was a plaque on the wall of the Ten Commandments, and in retrospect I can see where Mom exhibited the values of a Christian woman by the example she set for her three children. She didn't swear, smoke, or behave immorally. An eternal optimist, she worked hard and did everything in her power to expose us to arts and education, always encouraging us to reach for our dreams.

Nonetheless, we were still children confused by the divorce of our parents and the accompanying difficulties of living as welfare recipients on the edge of poverty.

Between my fear of the dark and emotionally repressed lifestyle, I survived grade school by creating a make-believe world. I had a dress-up collection that was the envy of all the neighborhood girls. Although money was always an issue, the Salvation Army Thrift Store was a treasure trove of joy for me as a youngster. I would navigate the aisles like a child with Glitter GPS to find the prom dress rack, where a quarter could buy a sublime gown and high heels went for a dime. I owned my first pair of stilettos when I was five, and although used and slightly scuffed, they were like precious glass slippers to me.

When I was in grade school I learned how to write. A new world opened up to me, as I had a natural inclination for writing to express myself. Drama also came naturally and in each play or skit I wrote I was always the princess, queen, damsel in distress, or heroine. Whatever the circumstances, I was always the one to be rescued by Prince Charming. Writing those fairy tale scenarios allowed me to create a world in which everything was perfect and safe, a place of eternal light and happiness where I never had to be afraid and the gallant knight in shining armor always showed up. Everyone lived happily ever after.

When I wasn't playing dress-up I spent many of my out-of-school hours watching old classic love stories on TV and reading romance magazines and novels. I began to pretend that I lived in a grown-up world of love, longing, beauty, and romance—long before I really knew what any of those things were. Without the love of an earthly father and no understanding of a heavenly Father, I was desperately seeking someone to fill that huge void.

Growing up, I saw how hard it was for my mom, raising three kids on her own. She was often lonely and frustrated, especially when money and housing issues reared their ugly heads. She cried a lot. I was convinced that Mom's loneliness, frustration, and fear were due to her need for a man to take care of her. I was sure that if she had a man—and we had a father— all would be right with the world. Therefore, I vowed that I was never going to be single. I was going to find a good man to take care of me, one that would care deeply for me and our children. We were going to own a house too—no one was going to raise our rent and threaten to evict us. I began keeping my "Mr. Right" list very early in life so that I wouldn't risk missing him when we met at last.

It was no surprise, then, that as a teenager I would drop out of school after the ninth grade, running away to get married when I met "Mr. Right." Except he wasn't. Only 15 years old, I wasn't a very good judge of character. What mattered in my mind was that this 18-year-old "man" represented security to me. I misinterpreted his obsessive need to control me as protection. The traits I initially saw as loving and warm quickly changed as I struggled for freedom within a dangerous relationship that soon became a painful prison. I now see how my damaged heart and soul caused my perception of him to be skewed.

The first time he hit me was shortly after we left the courthouse on the day we were married. In short order he went from being the love of my life to my abuser, jailer, kidnapper, rapist, and attempted murderer. I spent a horrific year married to him—a sadistic man whose extreme physical and emotional abuse almost killed me. Becoming pregnant at 16 was a defining moment that suddenly made my reality crystal clear. I was now responsible for the life of an unborn child and I had to keep this baby safe.

Escaping with my life, I returned to live with my mother where you buried the bodies under the house and everything was fine as long as you didn't talk about it—and so, we didn't.

Yet everything wasn't fine.

I had never been an overweight child but I gained a staggering 100 pounds during my pregnancy. My focus at that time was staying alive and protecting my unborn child. My mother gave me shelter and even though we moved several times to escape the wrath of this violent psychopath I had married, he always managed to find us. Afraid to leave the house I became reclusive, eating virtually from the time I woke up until I fell asleep. Food was the only comfort I could find. My mother only shook her head in sadness.

Every time I went to the clinic I would see a different obstetrician, and it wasn't until my ninth month that one of them actually connected the dots and read my chart, horrified that my weight had gone from 130 to 230 pounds in less than nine months.

In that retrospective wisdom that comes with time, I now see how excess weight kept me safe—protected. Eating was the only way I could avoid addressing the truth because the truth was utterly impossible for me to articulate. I had no words for the emotions I was feeling, but inside I was screaming.

This was when my struggle with food and weight began, when I developed one of the most destructive love/hate relationships I've ever known: my relationship with food. And this was the time when I came to believe unequivocally that if God existed it was certainly not in my world.

Can you recall any times in your childhood when food was your place of refuge? If so, write them in your journal.

Dealing with Demons

I was about 20 years old when a girl I met in my cosmetology class in Ohio introduced me to the world of prescription diet pills. These were commonly known as "appetite suppressants," but in reality were amphetamines, or speed. My four-year-old son and I had moved from my mom's apartment into our own place, and with the help of my "black beauty" pills, our apartment was spotless as I stayed up until the wee hours of the morning cleaning, polishing, scrubbing, waxing, organizing, and rearranging furniture. With these powerful little energy suppliers I felt invincible, able to accomplish countless tasks. I compensated for my debilitating fear of the dark by staying awake—working, cleaning, partying, or watching old movies.

Sleep did not come easily with amphetamines surging through my bloodstream. I didn't fall asleep so much as I collapsed from exhaustion or crashed and burned from too many late-night parties. Eventually, the same doctor who generously wrote prescriptions for the amphetamines began prescribing valium so I could get to sleep. A dangerous cocktail, especially in the hands of someone so emotionally and spiritually bankrupt.

With my appetite gone, I literally stopped eating. Soon, the weight I still carried from pregnancy began to melt off my body. It was the early seventies—the Age of Aquarius was being replaced by the disco beat and American psychologist Timothy Leary was advocating the therapeutic benefits of psychedelic drugs, particularly LSD and psilocybin mushrooms. I knew someone who could get both for me, and often did. Yet they did little to enlighten my world. I was running away from pain deep in my heart and soul, numbing my feelings with the busyness of life and the nonstop supply of speed, valium, mind-altering drugs, and pot.

Those of us battling the weight war know in our heart of hearts that our challenges are far more complicated than what we eat or don't eat. There's more going on emotionally than meets the eye. I'm not saying every person who struggles with weight issues is an emotional or psychological basket case but let's get real: If food has become our drug of choice to avoid our pain—if year after year is seeing diet after diet—then we have some issues to address.

Can you think of any issues you had in your teen years that you may not have addressed—or wish you had addressed differently? You might have to drill down to remember, but write down what comes to mind. Don't overthink this or censor yourself. Just write.

A Screeching Halt

One of the darkest periods of my adult life came about a year later. I had just begun to explore New Age spirituality, searching for meaning but coming up empty. Chris had entered kindergarten and I had just turned 21. I relished my independence but hated living alone. Still afraid of the dark, I would leave lights blazing all night and music played continuously whenever I was home.

Always looking over my shoulder for my abusive ex-husband to strike kept me edgy. My divorce didn't ensure freedom from violence, and restraining orders meant little to him. He had beaten me to within an inch of my life several times since our divorce and no one seemed able to help me. The longest he stayed in jail was two weeks, and when he was released he was more determined than ever to find me.

"Happy belated birthday to me," I said to myself that evening as I mixed my first drink, pouring a generous serving of vodka into the glass of chilled orange juice. By the end of the evening the entire fifth of alcohol would be gone, along with hundreds of pills—amphetamines, valium, and Quaaludes. It was a week or so after my twenty-first birthday, and I was feeling very old. Imagine that, feeling old at twenty-one! Yet the past five years had seemed like a lifetime.

Going back to school for my GED, working part time, raising my son, learning to drive, paying the bills—all of the day-to-day tasks that needed to be done were overwhelming for an adult, let alone a teenager. I may have felt alone but I wasn't entirely on my own. My mother helped a great deal, and without her I don't think I'd have made it. But that night I had grown weary of the constant struggle—I was tired of it all, including the weight problem I had developed when I got pregnant. The yo-yo dieting, starving, diet pills, mood swings, all of the responsibility—it was all so very much for me to handle.

I could no longer bury the feelings that churned inside me when I asked my mom to watch my son for the weekend, telling her I was going out of town. A friend suspected something was wrong and broke into my apartment, finding me in time to get me to the emergency room of a local hospital.

My suicide attempt brought me to my knees—not in prayer, but in utter hopelessness.

A mandatory three-day stay in the psychiatric ward of the hospital followed. This was my first introduction to professional counseling and the beginning of a climb out of hopelessness and into freedom that would take years.

Has there been a time in your past when you felt hopeless? When life wasn't worth living? If so, why? Write it down.

Unlocking the Truth

A counselor's astute questions in follow-up therapy, combined with writing exercises that often unlocked emotional doors I was unaware even existed, helped me begin to talk about things that weighed heavy on my heart—something I had never done in my life.

Therapy helped me begin to address the emotions I still carried as a battered wife, but far more important it also helped me confront my fear of the dark and my mother, bringing to light something I had always suspected deep inside my being.

The Secret Is Revealed

Shortly before my parents were divorced my mom had been hospitalized for a life-threatening bout with spinal meningitis during a time when my father was incarcerated. With no extended family available to care for us, my siblings and I were split up and sent to two temporary foster homes. My older sister was cared for by a loving woman, but my baby brother and I weren't so lucky.

When pressed for details, Mom shared a newspaper clipping she had kept for years, in which my infant brother and I were referred to as Jane Doe and Baby John Doe. In an instant, so much about my life suddenly made sense. As a child—a toddler—I was abused, molested, and locked in a closet under a stairwell by that foster parent—explaining my utter fear of the dark and nightmares. When I was found by authorities, my eyes were black and blue and swollen shut. I'd been severely beaten. Deeply traumatized, I screamed and cried for months afterward, prompting my mother to sleep at my bedside or hold me until I cried myself to sleep, an action that upset my father. It's been over a half century and I can still hear his voice to this day: "Leave her alone, Dolores. Quit babying her. She'll be okay."

I was never okay and neither were my parents. They divorced shortly thereafter.

It had been a brief period in physical time, a few weeks, but the mental and emotional damage lasted for decades.

I grew up afraid and screaming in the dark, and my brother spent years rocking himself to sleep. He had a habit of shaking his head back and forth on his pillow that drove us crazy but made perfect sense when you understood he had been neglected in his crib for days and was covered from head to toe in his own fecal matter when authorities found us. The constant shaking of his head had kept the flies from settling on his face and in his eyes and mouth.

Violated Boundaries

I've found that most people dealing with boundary-related weight issues are quite well-read when it comes to the latest diet trends. Countless weight loss books are sitting on the bookshelves of overweight men and women across the country. Most overweight Americans can recite verbatim a calorie, carbohydrate, or fat gram count, and are quite astute at knowing what they should and should not be eating. But ask them about the pain they carry in their hearts over a difficult or traumatic life-changing issue, or about a past filled with bitterness, unforgiveness, and hurt, and it's a different story.

Back in my teens, when I first began to seek comfort in food and recreational drugs, I was running from the pain of being a battered wife and the repressed memories of early childhood abuse. I never tried to understand the pathology of abuse, nor did I seek help to deal with the pain, anger, and fear that festered inside me. Oh, I knew I had been horribly abused—I wasn't in total denial—but the only way I knew to cope with it was to mirror how I'd been raised. I just figured if I didn't talk about it, it would go away. Alas, it did not go away. In fact, it only got bigger—along with my body.

Bernis Riley addresses the issue of violated boundaries often in her practice and says,

Abuse is a blatant violation of boundaries. It crosses all physical, mental, emotional, and psychological boundaries. But not only does abuse violate another person's boundaries, abuse causes a deep wounding of the soul. If left untreated, this wound becomes infected with anger, bitterness, resentment, fear, disappointment, and self-loathing. If you are a survivor of abuse, whether as a child or as an adult, counseling is recommended to help you find healing for your wounds of abuse.[6]

The Angry Truth

In her New York Times bestselling book *The Dance of Anger*, Dr. Harriet Lerner has helped countless women find clarity, calm, and a voice in their most difficult relationships. Anger is something we feel. It exists for a reason and always deserves our respect and attention. We all have a right to everything we feel—and certainly our anger is no exception.

> Anger is a signal, and one worth listening to. Our anger may be a message that we are being hurt, that our rights are being violated, that our needs or wants are not being adequately met, or simply that something is not right. Our anger may tell us that we are not addressing an important emotional issue in our lives, or that too much of ourselves—our beliefs, values, desires, or ambitions—is being compromised in a relationship. Our anger may be a signal that we are doing more and giving more than we can comfortably do or give. Or our anger may warn us that others are doing too much for us, at the expense of our own competence and growth. Just as physical pain tells us to take our hand off the hot stove, the pain of our anger preserves the very integrity of our self. Our anger can motivate us to say "no" to the ways in which we are defined by others and "yes" to the dictates of our inner self.[7]

My anger percolated for years after this painful discovery about my childhood, and I'm sorry to say that my relationship with my mother never fully healed. Refusing to talk anymore about what she referred to as "the incident," she returned the body to its grave under the house and retreated back to pretending it never happened—the safest place for her to exist.

I couldn't help but wonder how different my life may have been had I been able to talk with a professional child psychologist at any point in the years I was growing up. I could have avoided so many sleepless nights, terror-filled nightmares, and debilitating fears, night after night, month after month, and year after year. Instead, I formed a mind-body disconnect that would eventually lead to unhealthy thoughts, actions, and behaviors. It was here that my boundary confusion originated.

Chapter 9

Listening to the Hunger

Training ourselves to listen to our hunger may be one of the most challenging things we'll ever do. We've spent decades eating what we wanted when we wanted, or depriving ourselves of eating what we wanted when we wanted because we were on yet another diet.

Setting boundaries in any situation where they have been weak, nonexistent, or violated has to first become an intentional act before it can naturally become a healthy habit. Learning to listen to our hunger before we eat is a boundary that must be established on our road to finding freedom from the bondage of overeating or emotional eating.

The author of *Listen to the Hunger* agrees:

> As adults, what will happen to us if we stop hiding out in excess food and decide to face life? What happens when we choose to take our experiences head on without an anesthetic to dull the unavoidable pain? How do we become willing to feel, and what happens when we do? Listen to your hunger. Let it tell you what's really going on. The next time you have an urge to eat something when you just finished a meal an hour earlier, go behind the hunger and find out what's there.
>
> ...Some days there are many times when I have a feeling of emptiness and an urge to go looking for something to eat. If I give in to the urge, I don't learn anything about the hunger. If I stay with it, I often discover something I didn't know, a flash of insight that tells me what the hunger is really about.[1]

Learning to listen to what the hunger is really about isn't something we're taught. It's not a natural response when we want to eat. Heading for the refrigerator is the natural response.

Listening to the hunger causes us to ask what it is we're really craving. Understanding? Love? Acceptance? What emotions are welling up inside us when our first instinct is to push them back down with food? Fear? Anger? Worry? Many of us have been hiding our true emotions and needs for so long we haven't got a clue what they are. Remember, we have three primary needs: love, significance, and security. Are those needs being compromised, ignored, or violated?

I find that when I need to force myself to listen to the hunger, one of the issues—accusations, really—that often trips me up is a feeling that I'm not as smart or as bright as someone I'm comparing myself to. I don't *consciously* think I am stupid, but sometimes I *feel* stupid (especially if I begin the comparison game), and when that feeling bubbles to the surface the best way to silence it is to eat something. But if I stop long enough to drill down to the level where this feeling comes from, I can understand why I'm feeling it. The key here is stopping long enough to get beneath the surface.

For me, the bane of my existence in grade school was following an intellectually superior older sister. I think that's probably where the comparison game began. At the time I never thought of myself as stupid or inferior, but there was one teacher who always distinguished me as the "pretty sister" and Cheryll as the "smart sister." That distressed me to no end. Not that I minded being thought of as pretty, but I did mind being thought of as stupid. In fact, I minded it very much. And so I did what any deeply insecure and emotionally repressed schoolgirl would do. I made sure I showed everyone I met just how smart I really was, which landed me at the bottom of the popularity poll throughout my public school years. Actually, on some level I was okay with that because I found most girls were incredibly frustrating creatures to be around—always giggling, gossiping, and talking in riddles. They seldom said what they really meant and I thought most of them were rather silly.

Guys, on the other hand, were pretty straightforward. It was easier to talk to them and they didn't seem to play as many games—but for some crazy reason they always preferred the silly girls who did.

Go figure.

During the years after I had my son and struggled with my weight, I always felt smarter when I was heavier. Subconsciously, I equated being thin and pretty with being stupid. The inner conflict between thinking that guys liked silly girls but needing to be taken seriously as someone with a brain was something that took me years to sort out.

See what I mean by drilling down? There are a lot of layers to life.

Listening to our hunger is all about listening to our emotions. Remember, emotions are signals that tell us something about what is happening in our inner person. This can be very useful because we don't realize what's going on in our subconscious. That's why becoming more aware of our own emotions and emotional triggers can go a long way in helping us better understand what makes us tick—and what the hunger is *really* about.

Because of my past experiences there are times when someone may compliment me on how I look and there's a part of my brain that hears, "You are stupid and inferior." Subconsciously, this triggers a chain reaction of emotions that end up with me overeating because an inner voice is telling me that if I'm heavier I'll feel smarter, that people will take me seriously. When I go even deeper I come to a feeling of insecurity, a feeling that reminds me I'm a ninth-grade dropout and it's true, there are a lot of things I don't know.

Insane, isn't it? Absolutely—which is why the SANITY steps I'll present in this book are so helpful. The more I can intentionally stop and short-circuit those unhealthy and unproductive tapes from playing, the better.

It's critical to stop the initiating habit that keeps us from listening to the hunger in the first place, that makes us eat to avoid feeling and eat when we're not physically hungry.

Author and speaker Debra Peppers says,

> The easiest way for me to persevere in the midst of something that is difficult, or challenging, or when I'm emotionally attached is to simply "focus on focusing." This may involve little Post-it notes with motivators all over the house; it may mean asking my accountability partner (coach/mentor) to call me at certain intervals; or it sometimes involves writing a letter to myself and reading it over and over a thousand times.[2]

The next time you find yourself reaching for food when it isn't a meal-time or you've just eaten an hour or two ago, grab your notebook instead of eating and write down what it is that you're craving. Then ask yourself, "What is it I really *need*?" What happened just before you decided that food was the answer? Answer the following questions the author of *Listen to the Hunger* asks:

> The questions to ask yourself are, "What am I hungering for? What is my hunger really all about?" You have a craving, a feeling of emptiness. What will satisfy it? Maybe you used to think chocolate was the answer, but it didn't do the job. Your craving is an indication that you need something, but what? What is your hunger barometer telling you?[3]

When we've used food as an escape, as sedation, or as an answer to an unresolved question, listening to our hunger will most likely be a lifelong challenge—but it's a challenge we can overcome one day at a time when we decide to set healthy boundaries and live deliberately with SANITY.

Try to keep your notebook nearby and the next time you find yourself going to the refrigerator, pantry, or vending machine, or about to pull into a fast-food restaurant, I want you to deliberately stop yourself first and listen to what the hunger is *really* saying. Write it down. If your notebook isn't accessible use a piece of scratch paper or the back of an envelope, but write down what is happening and how it makes you feel.

Take a look at these examples below to see what I mean.

- I'm really not hungry, but my adult son just got fired from another job and *I'm afraid*...

- I'm really not hungry, but my boss has been loading me down with work and *I'm stressed*...

- I'm really not hungry, but my ex-husband has stopped paying child support and *I'm worried*...

- I'm really not hungry, but my financial situation is critical and *I'm desperate*...

- I'm really not hungry, but my project is due in a few weeks and *I'm insecure*...

It took me a while to learn there was so much more to my life than being thin and finding a man to protect me and provide for me, just as there is so much more to your life than whatever it is you're settling for. God has created us for a purpose. We all long to feel our lives have meaning—that our time on earth counts for something. There is a powerful big picture vision that exists inside each and every one of us—even if we've never acknowledged it or we're consistently burying it in empty calories and overeating. When we don't listen to the innermost cry of our hearts and spirits, what we're actually doing is "soul stuffing."

And enough is enough.

California, Here I Come

Although the pages in the scrapbook are brittle with age, the color remains vibrant on the dozens of clippings cut from magazines, catalogs, and newspapers, painstakingly preserved using photo-mount corners and printed captions. Every page documents not only my own career history, but history in the making in the world of fashion as well.

I'm in my mid-fifties as I write this book, and it's been a long time since I've paged through my old modeling portfolio from my years as one of the first plus-size models ever signed by the renowned Wilhelmina agency. It would be impossible to write about my journey of setting healthy boundaries with food and not walk down this particular memory lane. After all, it was a time when my weight, dress size, and measurements were discussed on a daily basis—a time when my entire life and livelihood revolved around my fuller figure, which was inextricably linked to food.

Another State, Another World

Following the lead of my younger brother and mother, I moved from Ohio to Southern California in the late 1970s, hoping to make a new start for my son and myself. And even more important, I was hoping to feel safe—hoping that my violent ex-husband wouldn't follow us across the country. Back home, I saw him in every shadow and every doorway. I had lived for years in constant fear for my life and the life of my son.

I enrolled in a local community college and secured part-time work as a hairdresser. As a single mother I was thankful for the additional aid of government assistance to make ends meet, but I knew it was only short-term. Being on welfare the rest of my life wasn't in my plan. Working in the entertainment world was my plan—preferably in the movies. Acting, writing, directing…I longed to do it all.

I'd grown up watching *The Wide World of Disney* every Sunday night, and the episodes where they actually featured Disneyland and the surrounding areas were my favorites. Back then I had no idea where Anaheim was, but I knew it was close to Hollywood and the Walk of Fame and Grauman's Chinese Theatre—and now here I was in Orange County, living the fairy tale—smack dab in the middle of it all! Somehow, I just knew that every Disneyland dream and Hollywood hope I ever had was going to come true.

We had been in California a short time when my mother happened to see the second issue of a glossy, high-quality fashion magazine featuring plus-size models.

"You could do this, Allison." Mom's eyes sparkled as she handed a copy of *Big Beautiful Woman* magazine to me. "You could be a fashion model." Eternally optimistic and hopeful, my mother was always my biggest cheerleader, encouraging me to reach for the stars.

Paging through the magazine, I felt a rush of excitement. At last, the one store that catered to us was about to lose its monopoly on providing clothes to women over size 14, as *Big Beautiful Woman* had now set the stage for plus-size fashions to be featured in a magazine that could go head-to-head with contemporary fashion magazines, with the exception that all of the models in the magazine were full-figured women. Back then, the only store that catered to us featured skinny models in their catalog.

I'd given up diet pills and was still struggling to lose the considerable weight I'd gained during my pregnancy years ago. Finding attractive and trendy clothes in larger sizes was always disheartening. However, since my little girl days of playing dress-up I had developed a creative flair when it came to fashion and didn't let the lack of clothes in my size stop me from dressing attractively. Between altering, sewing from scratch, and accessorizing, for years I'd lived the belief that a woman could be fashionable and full-figured. Just because we were heavy didn't mean we didn't care how we looked.

The editorial offices for *Big Beautiful Woman* were located in Los Angeles, and the fact that I lived in Southern California was a decided advantage. I was a hairdresser and makeup artist, which enabled me to change my look almost as quickly as I could change clothing, a big plus in the modeling industry at a time when hairdressers, makeup artists, and stylists were more the exception than the rule, and then typically reserved for high fashion shoots.

I'd never done anything like this, but in my early twenties, at a size 18 to 20, I figured that since they had just launched the magazine maybe I'd have a shot. What did I have to lose? A friend took photos for me and I mailed them to the *Big Beautiful Woman* offices.

In record time, I found myself in the Alfred Angelo design studios in Los Angeles, being fitted for one of the first plus-size wedding gowns in a new collection the famous designer was about to launch. In fact, I was appearing on the A.M. Los Angeles show that week wearing several of his gowns. The editor referred several potential models to the design house and I landed the job.

At that time modeling agencies didn't have full-figure models, so designers and manufacturers who were bold enough to join the cause and begin creating clothing for this market at first turned to *Big Beautiful Woman* for models—and to get their garments featured in the landmark magazine with an ever-increasing subscriber list. Today, every major modeling agency has an entire division for this category. Back then, I was the second plus-size model in the history of the legendary Wilhelmina Agency. New ground was being forged every day in an industry that didn't know quite what to do with models who had double-digit dress sizes. At times it was almost as though we were freaks in a carnival sideshow. But I was more than ready for the challenge and hit the ground running, as a two-year adventure into the world of plus-size modeling began.

In true Dickensian style, it was the best of times and the worst of times.

Full Figure, Empty Heart

Full-page ads for Levi-Strauss, Pendleton Knitwear, and Gloria Vanderbilt followed. In fact, Gloria Vanderbilt personally selected me as the model to introduce the very first line of designer jeans with zippers for plus-size women. You may read that and laugh, but it's true. It wasn't long ago that clothing over size 14 was limited to elastic waistband pants and shift-like muumuus.

Before long, every designer was throwing his or her hat into the ring.

Runway fashion shows, commercials, and an agent on Sunset and Vine in Hollywood were quite heady experiences for a girl from the projects of Cleveland, Ohio. Suddenly, my weight wasn't a hindrance. It was literally a "plus." Between school, modeling assignments, dating, and raising an increasingly strong-willed son, my life was busy—and exciting.

When a well-known swimsuit designer launched a line of suits for full-figured women it was history-making news in fashion, as was the company's decision to use plus-size models in their major ad campaign. I was selected as one of three. Shooting on the beach just south of Malibu, it truly was groundbreaking history. It felt good to be involved in something that was helping to increase the self-esteem of countless women. More and more major department stores began to devote floor space to plus-size women's wear, realizing we actually wanted to dress fashionably and had money to spend.

But it was only a matter of time before someone would see an easy target in the format of *Big Beautiful Woman* and lambaste this new trend. However, it didn't prepare me for the day a few months later when several of the swimsuit ad photos taken on the beach in Malibu showed up in a popular glossy men's magazine under the heading, *Can These Beached Whales Be Saved?* The accompanying story was equally harsh.

I felt violated, devastated, and humiliated.

Unable to articulate my emotions or address the situation in a healthy way, instead I found a doctor who would prescribe diet pills, doubled up on the dosage, and stopped eating, deluding myself that I'd be able to easily transition into the cadre of skinny models at Wilhelmina.

Not so.

It seemed that after I endured a considerable and hard-earned weight loss, I wasn't tall enough or pretty enough to be accepted into that incredibly competitive world. And although I was the thinnest I'd ever been in my adult life at 125 pounds, I still wasn't skinny enough.

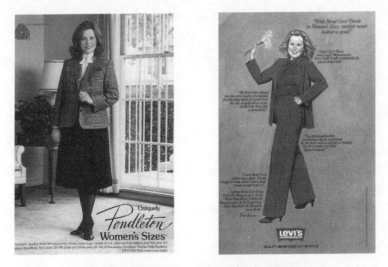

History making full page ads for plus-size fashion

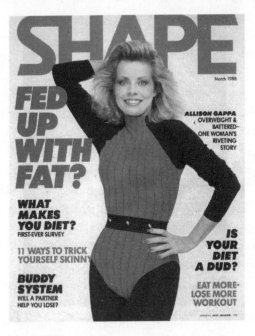

March 1988
My first magazine cover story. I starved myself
out of a job as a plus-size model. But my freelance writing career began. God had a plan.

My modeling career ended when I lost too much weight to qualify as a full-figure model. However, that lost weight didn't stay lost, and I would lose and gain and lose and gain hundreds of pounds over the following decade.

The Next Stage

I was determined to succeed no matter what the endeavor. On the outside I appeared confident, optimistic, and in control, and I'm sure most folks who knew me thought I had it all together. But on the inside I was lost and searching for love.

It was here that I earnestly began my spiritual search. I discovered New Age theology and developed my growing belief that we all carried a godlike (or goddess-like) power within ourselves. I changed my theology more often than I changed boyfriends (which was often), dabbling in tarot, Transcendental Meditation, Buddhism, mysticism, Taoism, Zen, and more.

To say I lacked spiritual balance would be an understatement.

After my modeling career ended I began what would become a lengthy career as a professional fund-raiser and special-event planner for nonprofit organizations. I also began to take my writing more seriously. I spent several years as the playwright-in-residence at a small theatre where three of my full-length plays were produced. My freelance writing career was moving along and I had been published in *Cosmopolitan*, *Ladies' Home Journal*, and *Shape* magazines. For *Shape* I appeared on the cover of an issue featuring my dramatic weight loss and my journey as one of the first plus-size models in the country (leaving out the part about starving myself and using diet pills, of course).

Today, I look at that cover of the woman wearing a blue exercise leotard with a cinched-in waist and a vacant, glassy-eyed stare and all I can remember is how hungry I was when the photo was taken. Hungry for food, hungry for faith, and hungry for love.

Still desperately searching for Prince Charming to rescue me, I would become engaged to and live with several different men over the course of the following years. Every broken engagement and shattered dream left me more emotionally crippled than the last. More than one abortion left additional scar tissue on my body, heart, and soul. I hit one dead end after another, never understanding that what I lacked was a Navigator who could help me chart a new course and stay on track.

I filled my days and nights with busy take-charge tasks, always on the move, always on a schedule, always following a list. I filled my soul with empty promises and emptier pursuits. The only constant thing in my life was my utter lack of healthy boundaries—with my son, the men in my life, and with food. There wasn't a time during this period when I ever accepted myself for who I was or when I felt contentment or peace in any area of my life. I numbed my pain with marijuana or food. The older my son got, the more rebellious he became. The more rebellious he became the more I tried to fix him—to change him. It was a vicious cycle of drama, chaos, crisis, and enabling, fueled by the emptiness I tried desperately to fill.

When I Began to Listen to the Hunger

The first time I stepped back and really listened to the hunger came at a time when everything around me was falling apart. It was the first time I made a conscious connection to the fact that I had developed a habitual pattern of filling the spiritual emptiness in my life with food and men, a pattern that never failed to cause rapid weight gain and almost always precipitated a major relationship crisis, which I was in at that moment.

For me, the habitual pattern was losing weight, searching for a man, finding a man, falling in love with the man, getting engaged to the man, moving in with the man, discovering I wasn't compatible with the man, and eventually breaking up with the man. Rapid weight gain always accompanied the last stage before breaking up, which would soon be followed by adopting another extreme diet where I would quickly lose weight and start the cycle all over again.

The only thing that changed over the years was the man.

Was it any wonder my son rebelled, finding his own acceptance in a culture of anarchy and drugs?

The Turning Point

I wasn't actively questioning my faith the night I found myself taking a less-than relaxing walk in my neighborhood of Orange, California. Frankly, I didn't understand the depth of the spiritual void in my life. That evening I was contemplating what steps I would need to take now that another engagement (my third in eight years) had been broken. I was only 35 years old. Less than an hour earlier, the final nail had been hammered into the coffin of another dying relationship. Because the property was in my now-ex-fiancé's name, I had to move from the home we had shared. "As soon as possible," he said as I stormed out of the house.

The financial ramifications of this breakup began to compete with my broken heart. I had really loved this man—or so I thought. Thoughts of how I would cope with the increasing responsibility and time demands of my job while trying to find somewhere to live overwhelmed me. I loved my work in nonprofit development, but my inability to set healthy boundaries affected virtually every area of my life. As I took on more and more responsibility at work the level of stress grew proportionally.

Topping it all off was the main subject that began the argument with my fiancé, or rather ex-fiancé, earlier that evening. My son had just been picked up and incarcerated in the county juvenile detention facility. He would be 18 in a few weeks—a legal adult—and if he continued down the path he was on the severity of the consequences would increase. Since he had turned 13 and began running with the Huntington Beach punk community, the drama, chaos, and crisis surrounding his life became more and more difficult—and costly—for me to handle. His rebellion caused my heart such anguish and it seemed no matter what I did to try to help it was only temporary. Nothing seemed to work. (And nothing *would* work until I learned the difference between helping and enabling and started setting healthier boundaries in my own life and in the relationship with my son—a lesson that was still years away and is told at length in my first Setting Boundaries® book, *Setting Boundaries with Your Adult Children*.)

In addition to arguing about the situation concerning my son, we had also argued about my weight, which was once again creeping back up the scale, a typical syndrome whenever a relationship failed to meet the needs of my heart and soul. Actually, "creeping" isn't a good word choice. It was more like leaping, as I'd probably put on a good 50 pounds in less than six months. Nothing fit me anymore, and I had to once again unpack my boxes of "fat clothes" so I'd have something to wear.

"If you really loved me my weight wouldn't be an issue!" I'd cried earlier, pulling clothes from the box I'd retrieved from the back of the closet. "It's who I am on the inside that counts!"

Does this sound at all familiar? It's an argument many of us have with loved ones when we live on the weight cycling diet treadmill.

While there is truth to the fact that God calls us to love and we shouldn't judge based on appearance—and I know firsthand the bitter truth about how quickly people pass judgment on someone because of their weight—the truth is, internal struggle can often masquerade as external weight. No matter how much we argue that we're the same person on the inside no matter what we weigh, I'm afraid that isn't usually the case.

My ongoing search for Prince Charming once again left me brokenhearted. All I had ever wanted was someone to love me, to make me feel safe and special. Three needs: love, significance, and security. But I had expected so much from the men in my life—to fix my broken soul, mend my son, fill me, complete me, protect me, and keep me safe. I wanted them to make me feel special, significant, as though I were a princess. Yet there was no way an earthly love could ever give me everything I needed. Those needs couldn't be met in any earthly relationship, but only in a relationship with the Father, Son, and Holy Spirit.

I fought back tears as I continued to walk and tried to think. I was at a loss about what I should do first, and frankly, my New Age "goddess within" strength was worthless. In fact, I was *not* strong. I was utterly and completely lost and I didn't know where to turn. As for faith, I always came up empty, no matter which New Age religion I studied or tried to incorporate into my life. I lived as if my search for metaphysical meaning could be some kind of salvation in and of itself, yet it never was.

Somehow I would manage to survive. I always did, even if each transgression left me lonelier and emptier. *Soon there will be nothing left of my heart*, I thought sadly.

It was then I noticed activity around me as people were parking and getting out of cars nearby and going in to the neighborhood church. I had often stopped what I was doing to listen to the bells of this church as they chimed strangely familiar hymns from my childhood days in Vacation Bible School. *It must be a funeral or a meeting or something*, I thought, never imagining a church would have a weekday evening service.

Suddenly, I crossed the street on legs that were not my own, reading the sign on the wall: Wednesday Evening Service, 7:00 PM. Could I go inside if I was not a member? Would they let me in? I felt so ignorant. Then, as my mind shifted into gear, telling me all the reasons I shouldn't go inside, my legs once again developed a mind of their own, virtually propelling me up the steps and through the doors.

A sign with an arrow pointing to the balcony beckoned me. As I walked up the steps I worried, *Will someone come and throw me out, knowing I don't belong here?* I had no idea what I was doing, where I was going, or what to expect. I was quite literally not in control of my actions as I climbed the stairs.

Discovering the Empty Vessel

As I walked under the arched doorway and entered the balcony, it was as though I had stepped from an air-conditioned car or building and out into the warm summer air, a feeling that took my breath away. A "whoosh" seemed to envelop me, leaving me a little weak, a little disoriented. There was no one else in the balcony, adding to my concern that I was probably somewhere I shouldn't be, but which allowed me to gasp in awe as I gazed at a sanctuary straight out of an epic film. With an immense arched ceiling with gold leaf edging, gleaming dark woodwork and pews, and breathtaking stained-glass windows, this building was a work of art, and I could appreciate the majesty of it all.

Being alone also allowed me to fall back unnoticed into one of the pews as I looked toward the pulpit and saw the statue of Jesus with outstretched arms, looking right at me. If I live to be one hundred years old I will still recall that moment. He was staring at me. Jesus was staring at *me*. Hot tears fell down my cheeks as emotions I couldn't explain filled my heart and soul.

When the pastor began to speak it was as though his message was for me alone. A message of being lost, without direction, without hope, without faith—and how that was not God's plan for my life. He talked about love—God's love for us—God's love for me, no matter how badly I had sinned or fallen short. He talked of how we needed only to ask the Lord Jesus Christ to come into our heart and He would be there—just like that.

What was happening to me? Why was I sitting in a strange church crying like a baby? *Thank God I am alone up here*, I thought, *or they would be carting me off to a loony bin.* Then it hit me. Yes! Thank God! That was why I was here. That was why He had led me up the steps and into my own private balcony—to acknowledge Him, to thank Him for all He had done and was about to do in my life and in my son's life. He opened my eyes, touched my soul, and gave me something I had lacked for far too long: hope, faith, and love.

At that moment I understood that I would never be alone or unloved. That I was inextricably, inexplicably connected to the God of the universe.

I couldn't see through the tears flowing nonstop from somewhere deep within my soul, but I could see in another way, more clearly than I had in a long, long time. Instead of looking through the eyes of one in fear, bondage, and sin, I was suddenly seeing from the wonderful vantage point of freedom and redemption. It was a transcendent experience that sparked a new perspective of possibility in my soul. It was as though the ground shifted under me and I suddenly turned a corner and life as I had known it was over.

My walk with the Lord started that day, a day that forever changed the course of my life.

> Though you have made me see troubles,
> many and bitter,
> you will restore my life again;
> from the depths of the earth
> you will again bring me up (Psalm 71:20 NIV).

Renewal Awaits

True to His Word, God restored my life and brought me up from the depths.

That's not to say life was suddenly filled with roses and sunshine. I had begun an amazing U-turn in my life, but on the home front I still had a broken heart to deal with, finances to sort out, a son in jail, and tremendous job stress—not to mention I still needed to find somewhere to live. *Maybe living together isn't the best way to do things*, I found myself saying for the first time in my life. It would be the first of many convictions I would eventually have that contradicted worldly lies I had believed for so long.

Where before my self-centered search had been focused on finding the "goddess within," this time I was searching for the one true God. This time I came face-to-face with a God who loved me for who I was—no matter what I had done. I was special in His eyes and that fact changed my heart—and my life.

New Direction

When I began to put God first, amazing things started to happen. The world opened up to me in ways I could never have imagined. Within a week I had secured an apartment and moved. I began attending church and reading my Bible and every Christian testimony I could get my hands on. More importantly, the Lord understood my need and, keeping His promise, began to send people into my life to lend me support, guidance, and strength. I was beginning to understand what it meant to belong to a family of believers.

This sudden spiritual illumination didn't make my life perfect, but it was a life of healing and hope, a life of new perspective and promise where before there had been empty desolation that I often filled with food and destructive relationships.

My son, however, was unwilling to embrace my newfound faith. When he turned 18 and was released from the juvenile detention center, free to chart his own course, he took off for parts unknown. This was the first of many seasons in which I had no idea where he was or if he was even alive, when I began to fear every late-night phone call. For the first time, I began to pray for his salvation and his safety, praying that one day he too would make a U-turn toward God. Still, I grieved the damage my foolish choices had done to him in his formative years, and it was often grief that increasingly fueled my own enabling choices as the years went by, even as I grew in my faith.

My earthly relationships were never going to make me complete. It took me a long time to understand I had been looking in all the wrong places for true love.

Define the Hunger

I've shared this part of my story with you because it was the first time I drilled down beneath the surface of the pain in my life and made a conscious connection that I was using food to fill more than my stomach. And without the power of the Holy Spirit that connection would never have happened.

It's been said there is a God-shaped place in every heart that only God can fill. And whether you're a seasoned saint or a new believer, there are times in life when our relationship with God isn't the priority it needs to be. It's often during those times that we get caught up in the insanity that characterizes difficult situations—and difficult people. Times when we're not listening to what the hunger is really telling us.

Clearly, I hadn't been good at developing long-term relationships over the years. I knew nothing of boundaries—healthy or otherwise—and I repeatedly jumped on the same catastrophic carousel ride when it came to relationships with men—looking always for protection, safety, security, and love. A walking, talking, human blob of needs and insecurities, the only thing I seemed capable of accomplishing was drastically losing weight, falling in love, gaining weight, falling out of love, and then starting the cycle all over again.

But in reality—was it really love I was falling into time after time? Or something altogether different? What unresolved needs were these relationships filling? More important, how could I short-circuit the habit of using food to bring comfort when relationships didn't fulfill those needs?

Critical Questions

Healthy people in healthy relationships know what their needs are and can address them calmly and rationally at the point where the need is making itself known. They don't turn to something else to bury the need.

On the other hand, unhealthy people in unhealthy relationships have developed the habit of ignoring their needs, burying them instead under the false comfort of food.

As we strive to listen to the hunger, we must ask ourselves four critical questions.

1. What am I really craving?
2. What would it take to satisfy my soul?
3. What emotion is being sedated when I eat when I'm not physically hungry?
4. How can I break the habit of putting food into my mouth and intentionally address what I really need?

The Key to Listening

When the numbers on my scale increase, it's usually because my focus on God has decreased and my life is out of balance. Somewhere along the line I've neglected my spiritual Slice-of-Life section in the Balance Pie, and the results of that neglect are usually rather quickly evident.

Listening to our hunger often means addressing painful emotions or difficult situations, and when we've developed the habit of using food as a substitute to addressing painful emotions or difficult situations, it's going to take supernatural power to give us courage and strength—and that comes from God alone. Being able to listen to our hunger begins with listening to God. They are inextricably connected.

It's a significant accomplishment when we're able to say "Stop" as we reach for food when we aren't physically hungry, to recognize that something else is going on and, at that point of recognition, being able to catch our destructive thoughts and actions and actually stop.

> We destroy every proud obstacle that keeps people from knowing God. We capture their rebellious thoughts and teach them to obey Christ (2 Corinthians 10:5).

Chapter 10

The Conviction of Sin

"Are you sure we are doing the right thing?" I asked my fiancé as we signed the leasing papers. We were moving into a large apartment high on the hill in Yorba Linda, California.

"Of course we are," Tim said lovingly as he kissed my cheek. "We're together all the time anyway. It doesn't make much sense to pay rent on two places. We'll save money this way—surely God will understand the financial aspect. Plus, we're getting married. It's not like we're just planning on living together."

Justification started early in our relationship, and slipping into my old way of life was at first incredibly easy to do. Living with a man out of wedlock was not new to me, but doing so as a Christian *was* new to me, and this time for all of the worldly justification, something didn't seem quite right.

"Allison, it's clear your mind is made up," my pastor said gently to me when I told him of our plans. His unconditional love spoke volumes to this new Christian.

"I can't tell you what to do or not to do, but I can tell you what Jesus would want you to do and what Scripture says about premarital relations, and I can pray for the Holy Spirit to convict you about this choice—about the real truth."

As a new believer I was having a tough time understanding this enigma of the Holy Spirit. Was it a voice you heard in your head? Some divine inspiration that came from the clouds, filling you with an immediate sense of knowledge and wisdom? If so, what did I have to do to get Him to talk to me? I would have appreciated a more vocal directive.

Living with Tim during our engagement seemed right from a logical perspective. Surely there were allowances being made from what was inappropriate in biblical times to the accepted standards of *this* century.

I had met Tim not long after coming to know Christ, and felt certain he was an answer to my prayers. It was love at first sight and we were soon engaged. Tim began attending classes at my church and was baptized by the same pastor who had led me to the Lord a few months earlier. This was the pastor who was now telling me that what Tim and I were doing was wrong in God's eyes. But not just wrong. According to him it was a sin.

Clinging to Old Habits

In an earlier chapter I wrote about the importance of nurturing our relationship with God. The more involved we are in this deeply personal heart relationship, the more we learn about the wisdom, power, and glory of God. As our Christian faith grows, so, too, does our understanding of God's character and the indefinable certainty of His Word. Clearly, there is a standard for life as a Christian.

But oh, how we battle to hang on to old habits. How great is our obstinacy! Just listen to Oswald Chambers, author of the classic devotional *My Utmost for His Highest*.

> There is any amount of weakness in us all, but deep down there is red-handed rebellion against the authority of Jesus Christ—I'll be damned before I yield. Don't take a political view of things that go beyond science. At bottom, sin is red-handed mutiny that requires to be dealt with by the surgery of God—and he dealt with it on Calvary.[1]

Red-handed rebellion and mutiny. Oswald Chambers was describing me to a T in my early walk with the Lord, when I tried to justify my sinful behavior as a morally acceptable standard for modern times.

Truthfully, we need to get right—and stay right—with God.

The "getting right" part is relatively easy. This occurs when we admit we are sinners and ask for God's forgiveness and mercy, accepting the Lord as our Savior. It's the "staying right" component that often trips us up. Learning to discern what is good and right and just—and what is sin—according to God's Word, and walking in one while retreating from the other, is not an easy calling.

When Did We Get So Open-Minded That Our Brains Slipped Out?

The subject of absolute truth and morality has become the topic of great debate as biblical interpretation has become skewed and as the value system of our society has shifted.

Leslie Vernick says, "We do what we do not because of what has happened *to* us, but because of what is *in* us."

What is it that is *in* us? One word—"sin." We are in desperate need of a national, even a global U-turn—a U-turn revival where people turn away from their *sin*. But that, my friend, cannot happen until we know what sin is. And therein lies the problem.

The definition of sin is living independently of God's standard—knowing what's right, but choosing what's wrong. However, it's not the definition of sin but the *interpretation* of sin that confuses us.

Whose interpretation of sin do we use?

Who dictates what is right?

The Bible says, "Remember, it is sin to know what you ought to do and then not do it" (James 4:17).

"One man's sin is another man's salvation," I once heard. *"It's a free country. Who am I to judge?"* some say. We tolerate sins expressly forbidden by the Bible and ignore the commands of Jesus. We have become utterly nonjudgmental, refusing to set ethical or moral boundaries for fear of being considered politically incorrect. Why do we accept without argument the shifting tide of tolerance for all things? We've become so open-minded that our brains have slipped out!

Perhaps I'm so saddened by the sin our country lives in because I know it so well. I know from experience how devastating its effects can be. For decades I felt dirty, ashamed, used, empty, and lost—all of which fed my food addiction. I spent so much time focusing on finding a man to protect and provide for me, and on the problems of my adult child, involved in the ongoing crisis, chaos, and drama in his life, that I neglected my own emotional, psychological, financial, and spiritual health.

I didn't know it, but I ached for something only God was able to give me. Forgiveness, redemption, salvation, peace, joy, hope, healing, and most of all love. My life began when I turned toward God. It was God who convicted me of the sin in my life and God who gave me the strength to set healthy boundaries and find sanity. He can do the same for you.

Could it be that in *not* setting healthy boundaries we are actually sinning? Could enabling be a sin? Could rescuing our adult children from walking their own Damascus road journeys be a sin? Is it a sin when we give our hard-earned money to an addicted adult child? In our well-meaning desire to make things easier for our adult children, is it a sin that we have robbed them of the tools they need to become responsible and productive adults?

Could it be a sin when we allow a spouse or ex-spouse, in-law, boss, coworker, family member, neighbor, or friend to distract us from our priority relationship with God—stealing our peace and robbing us of joy? Is it a sin when we don't guard our own hearts and consistently allow people to overstep boundaries and hurt us? Is it a sin to overeat? To neglect our bodies?

The last thing we need when our hearts are breaking is someone pointing a finger at us. We feel guilty enough as it is—believe me, I know. But when will the scales fall away from our eyes, allowing us to see the part we have played in the story of our lives? When will we start to make sane choices that will address the sin in our lives and help us change?

Experiencing the fullness of a life lived in fellowship with a loving, personal God requires sacrifice and obedience on our part. It's the obedience part that often keeps us distanced from experiencing God in all His fullness, glory, and grace.

Clinging to Old Habits

In my mind living with Tim seemed logical, but in my heart it was another story. As the weight of conviction began to weigh heavy on my spirit, I was beginning to understand that a relationship with Jesus is not one-sided. I had taken the gift of salvation and redemption willingly, with an open heart. But somehow I began to think that the most important aspect of Christianity was to confess our sins and get forgiveness and eternal life. And while that is an important aspect, Jesus offers us far more than forgiveness. We now have a personal and intimate relationship with Him in which He calls us His child.

For the first time in my life I had a Father who loved me unconditionally. Instead of treating Him with love and respect I adjusted His wise teaching to suit me, not only ignoring the relationship that had changed my life but the words the Holy Spirit was clearly trying to speak to me.

He got my attention when my pants ripped.

No time to eat, have to run errands on my lunch break, just a part of life, I thought to myself as I grabbed my purse, all but flying out the door of my office. Unlocking the car door, I tossed my purse in the back and quickly slid into the front seat to the accompanying sound of *Rrrriiiiiipppp!* I'd ripped out the entire back seam of my pants.

Earlier that day I had wriggled into the Carole Little designer pants thinking, *Wow, these are really tight.* But covered by the matching, loose-fitting tunic I figured I'd be okay—who would see?

Well, my fiancé, who had spent the night at my place, had seen, and commented (not too subtly) on my weight that very morning. I had stomped out of my apartment wearing the too-tight pants and vowing not to speak to Tim until he apologized for being so rude.

But he was right; I had gained weight over the months since we met and fell in love—almost 40 pounds, to be exact. I could no longer hide behind loose-fitting clothes; nothing fit anymore. I was miserable when I was supposed to be happy. I was marrying a handsome doctor, we were moving into a lovely hillside apartment, and we were both new Christians—what more could I ask for?

Someone who accepts me for who I am, I thought angrily as I let Tim's words about my weight gain sink into my heart. The more I thought about it the more I realized how obsessed he was with physical looks. He went to the gym every day, not just a few times a week. I, on the other hand, was not big on exercise.

I began to get angrier and angrier at Tim, neglecting to look into my own heart and soul at the root of the problem. I was justifying sin and returning to old habits that had only brought me emptiness and pain in my past.

When would I learn?

The intimate relationship between a husband and wife is one of God's most precious gifts. Unfortunately, in these modern times it's also a boundary we have grown to view as an acceptable one to cross.

In her *Counseling Through Your Bible Handbook*, June Hunt has much to say regarding the lifelong commitment of marriage and the benefits of premarital counseling. "In order to build a strong foundation for marriage, learn as much as possible about yourself, your future mate, and God's will for marriage...before you tie the knot."[2] She goes on to say:

> A couple who wants to experience the maximum out of marriage needs to look at God's original design for the marital relationship. The Bible tells us that marriage is to reflect the sacrificial love that Christ has for His bride, the church. Although the backgrounds of a husband and wife may be different and expectations may differ, they can develop unity of heart through mutual submission and godly respect for one another.[3]

God's original design didn't include test-driving a marriage before making the commitment. My own history should have been proof enough, but I convinced myself that this time it was different. After all, we were both Christians and planning to marry. Some habits really are hard to break, especially when popular opinion supports you. Had I known the Six Steps to SANITY at the time, this would most definitely have been the time to stop, listen to God's guidance, and trust the voice of the Spirit. He was speaking loud and clear! I was just choosing not to listen. Thankfully, He wasn't giving up on me yet!

Seeking Help to Turn from Sin

So there I was, sitting in my car at the stoplight, crying, with the back end of my pants ripped out. Not a pretty picture. I couldn't stop crying tears of anger over ripping my pants, over Tim's words that morning, over the seesaw of weight losses and gains, and over the deep, unsettling feelings I was having in my soul about the entire relationship. Hadn't I learned anything since giving my heart to the Lord? Everything welled up inside as my tears turned to sobs—drowning out the sounds of irate motorists behind me, honking for me to move.

Then suddenly, as though God stepped in and orchestrated it, a commercial came on the car radio for a Christ-centered treatment center.

"Does the pain in your life seem too much to bear?"

Was this fellow talking to me?

"Does a food, alcohol, drug, or relationship addiction have you in bondage?"

My ears perked up.

"Then call this number right away!" said the announcer, rattling off an easy-to-recall number.

I repeated the number over and over again as sobs literally wracked my body. This wasn't a normal crying spell (if you've had any kind of emotional breakdown you know what I mean). Something was seriously wrong and I was afraid. I took my foot off the brake, accelerated quickly, and pulled over to the curb, throwing the car into park and then grabbing change from my purse.

Getting out of the car and practically running to a phone booth (this was before cell phones were commonplace), I dropped coins into the phone and dialed the number.

I had received a glorious gift the day I accepted Jesus Christ as my Lord and Savior. I knew that truth in every fiber of my being. Yet I felt as though a part of me was dying that day as I called the residential treatment center from the claustrophobic phone booth. My emotions ran amuck. I was confused, angry, guilty, and ashamed as I poured out my heart to the operator who answered my call.

"It's going to be okay, honey," she gently said. "Where are you?"

"I don't know where I am. I'm lost…" My throat knotted up as I gave voice to the gut-wrenching truth. Despite the euphoria I had felt since accepting the Lord, there was still an incredibly damaged little girl living inside of me who was desperately and frightfully lost—and no amount of food or earthly relationships could make her better. I was still using food and a man to avoid my emotions—to avoid addressing my needs. I wasn't being honest with myself or God.

I had claimed 2 Corinthians 5:17 as a foundational rock early in my faith walk. "Therefore, if anyone is in Christ, he is a new creation: the old has gone, the new has come!" And although the new had indeed come in many ways, I was still struggling as I sat on the fence between two worlds. As I began to feel the pain of Holy Spirit conviction, I realized there was much I still had to do on my journey to experience true freedom.

The time had come for me to choose on which side of the fence I wished to live—in the Word or in the world? How long could I justify sin?

It was no coincidence that the treatment center was just a few miles from where I stood. And so it was I came to a fork in the road in my life, a fork that led me to check myself into a Christian psychiatric facility on my lunch hour. I remained there for the next 30 days.

A part of me *was* dying that day—and *it needed to*—before I could fully grasp the depth and power of God's love for me.

Once again Oswald Chambers speaks directly to the heart of this issue.

> When once the real touch of conviction of sin comes, it is hell on earth—there is no other word for it. One second of realizing ourselves in the light of God means unspeakable agony and distress; but the marvel is that when the conviction does come, there is God in the very center of the whole thing to save us from it.[4]

And save me from it He did, as I began the hard work of building boundaries that had never existed and repairing those that had long ago crumbled. As Cloud and Townsend teach,

> God's desire is for you to know where your injuries and deficits are, whether self-induced or other-induced. Ask him to shed light on the significant relationships and forces that have contributed to your own boundary struggles. The past is your ally in repairing your present and ensuring a better future.[5]

The Fog Lifted

It took three days of around-the-clock care before I exhausted my soul of the tears I felt safe enough to shed. True to His Word, God sent loving people to bind up my wounds. Christian counselors and therapists prayed for me while physicians and nurses monitored my vital signs, administered medication, and kept fluids flowing into my veins.

When at last I was able to come up from the fog, I entered the general population on the ward and began the hard work of piecing together the fractured fragments of my life. From sunup until sundown, every waking moment was spent in individual therapy, group therapy, drama therapy, or prayer. With the support and encouragement of a gifted team of caregivers, I was processing my entire life with the sole purpose of finding inner healing and peace.

We discussed my childhood, including the abuse and molestation I'd experienced as a little girl, and the years of fear after that had gripped my heart and soul. We talked about what it was like having an emotionally absent mother, and how that affected my entire life. We discussed my teenage marriage and the brutal abuse at the hands of a man who was supposed to love, honor, and cherish me—the Prince Charming I had searched for my entire life. We talked about my son, how hard it had been to raise him on my own, the mistakes I had made and the guilt I felt. We talked about the many broken relationships and broken hearts that had left me feeling alone and empty. I confessed sin after sin, laying everything at the foot of the cross.

Drama therapy sessions in our group environment left me emotionally drained. I often cried for days after these sessions and tears became both a cleansing agent for washing away the last vestiges of painful memories while also nurturing the seeds of hope that were forming in their place.

The Truth About Turning to Food

All the while I was being encouraged to look at how my weight—and food—had played an integral part in my life and my choices. It was here I discovered the valuable tool of writing down my thoughts, feelings, and emotions—without censoring myself. At the treatment center I came to see that prayer properly applied was the antibiotic that healed open sores and brought inner peace.

Clearly, the Lord had brought me to His side a year previous to pave the way for this place in time. He had brought me to a place where I would find safety in the arms of professionals—people who could help me on the journey through my pain and deliver me on the other side, ready for the next stage of my new life in Christ. This healing journey was the second time I felt born again, and I can tell you beyond a shadow of a doubt that I would not have been able to maintain my 120-pound weight loss all these years after weight loss surgery had I not first dealt with these deeply personal and unbelievably painful issues.

During my month-long stay in the hospital, I began to see for the first time the entire big picture of my life. It was here I first began to understand the meaning of boundaries—a totally foreign concept to me. I saw how my past fit together, how I had come to this place in time—and I suddenly knew I could be free from the emotional bondage that had once held me captive. The Holy Spirit began to convict me to look at the sin in my life, past and present. I was being changed from the inside out and it hurt like nothing I'd ever before experienced.

The Sin of Gluttony

Everybody in the world, in every culture, has known that overeating is bad for us. From the ancient Greeks to the modern age, we have been told to be moderate in our eating. In the Judeo-Christian tradition on which our society was founded, overeating isn't just bad for us, it is bad, period. As in morally wrong. However, in our modern consume-consume-and-consume-some-more culture, gluttony isn't a sin, it's a virtue. We're encouraged to eat, and eat more, and eat a big dessert on top of that. We worship at the altar of the all-you-can-eat buffet.

Much like the transcendent experience I had in the church when I first connected to God, the awareness of the effects our sinful natures have on our lives ushered in a transformational revelation that began to change my life. The Word of God says:

> So I say, let the Holy Spirit guide your lives. Then you won't be doing what your sinful nature craves. The sinful nature wants to do evil, which is just the opposite of what the Spirit wants. And the Spirit gives us desires that are the opposite of what the sinful nature desires. These two forces are constantly fighting each other, so you are not free to carry out your good intentions. But when you are directed by the Spirit, you are not under obligation to the law of Moses.
>
> When you follow the desires of your sinful nature, the

The Conviction of Sin

results are very clear: sexual immorality, impurity, lustful pleasures, idolatry, sorcery, hostility, quarreling, jealousy, outbursts of anger, selfish ambition, dissension, division, envy, drunkenness, wild parties, and other sins like these. Let me tell you again, as I have before, that anyone living that sort of life will not inherit the Kingdom of God.

But the Holy Spirit produces this kind of fruit in our lives: love, joy, peace, patience, kindness, goodness, faithfulness, gentleness, and self-control. There is no law against these things!

Those who belong to Christ Jesus have nailed the passions and desires of their sinful nature to his cross and crucified them there. Since we are living by the Spirit, let us follow the Spirit's leading in every part of our lives. Let us not become conceited, or provoke one another, or be jealous of one another (Galatians 5:16-26).

Forgiveness of Sin

As a little girl I had played dress-up, and make-believe was the creative avenue I took when loneliness, fear, emptiness, or hopelessness filled my soul. I had created a fantasy life to deal with the early abuse I had suffered as a child at the hands of a foster parent—it was how I survived. I went from that young girl playing dress-up to a teenage wife, believing I had actually found the Prince Charming who would rescue me. When it became obvious I had made a horrible mistake, I could no longer use the escape of my childhood to fill the emptiness in my soul. I turned instead to food, and then to other relationships. Over time I graduated to drugs, alcohol, socializing, overworking, and materialism. Eventually I immersed myself in New Age theology.

It took decades of being lost before I opened my heart to the healing power of the Holy Spirit and accepted the Lord as the Supreme Navigator of my life. Then it took a month in a residential treatment facility to begin fitting all the pieces together and start doing the necessary work to adjust my life to God, a task Henry Blackaby says could be the greatest difficulty believers will ever have:

If you want to be a disciple—a follower—of Jesus, you have
no choice. You will have to make major adjustments in your
life to follow God. Following your Master requires adjustments in your life. Until you are ready to make any adjustment necessary to follow and obey what God has said, you will
be of little use to God. Your greatest single difficulty in following God may come at the point of adjustment.[6]

Much of the necessary adjustment work I had to do revolved around
sin and forgiveness.

Like Joseph in the Old Testament, who forgave his brothers for sell-
ing him into slavery, I forgave the foster parents who hurt me, the ex-
husband who abused me, and the men in my life who turned out not to
be Prince Charming. I forgave the mother who didn't get me the help I so
desperately needed as a child, and who in her inability to express her own
emotions had taught me to ignore mine. I forgave myself for the choices
I made that had taken me down countless dead-end streets.

And I knew beyond any doubt that Jesus forgave me.

I didn't marry Tim. We broke up while I was still in treatment.

It was the last time I lived with someone out of wedlock.

There is nothing attractive about the Gospel to the natural
man; the only man who finds the Gospel attractive is the man
who is convicted of sin. Conviction of sin and being guilty of
sins are not the same thing. Conviction of sin is produced by
the incoming of the Holy Spirit because conscience is promptly
made to look at God's demands and the whole nature cries out,
in some form or other, "What must I do to be saved?"[7]

The Cost of Conviction

Yes, when we give our lives to Jesus there is a cost, but it is a small price
to pay for the rewards of a heart relationship with Someone who will meet
all of our needs for love, significance, and security. To know we will never
be alone, afraid, or empty again—that our dependence and obedience will
be rewarded with a life of purpose and meaning—that is worth the price
of any adjustment needed.

The adjusting is to a Person. You adjust your life to God. You adjust your viewpoints to be like His viewpoints. You adjust your ways to be like His ways. After you make the necessary adjustments, He will tell you what to do next to obey Him. When you obey Him, you will experience Him doing through you something only God can do.[8]

Ask God to bring you to a place of adjustment, to a place where you can be free of the bondage that food, dieting, or weight has had on you. Pray for Holy Spirit conviction about the things in your life keeping you from experiencing that intimate heart relationship with the Lord.

A Word About Satan

A master of deception, Satan has used our experiences to build a fortress of lies in our thinking. Satan is first and foremost a deceiver, and we must do everything possible to remove him from power in our life. When we sin, we hand over to Satan a poisonous weapon that he will eagerly use against us. It's critical that as we strengthen our bond with the Lord Almighty, we ask Him to reveal the sin in our life and we repent accordingly.

We are made right with God by placing our faith in Jesus Christ. And this is true for everyone who believes, no matter who we are. For everyone has sinned; we all fall short of God's glorious standard. Yet God, with undeserved kindness, declares that we are righteous. He did this through Christ Jesus when he freed us from the penalty for our sins (Romans 3:22-24).

Chapter 11

Food Sense and Sensibilities

It's difficult and painful when we have people in our lives we care about who don't care about themselves, people who abuse their bodies with drugs, alcohol, nicotine, and more. I'm the mother of a drug-addicted adult child (in recovery and drug free!), and I know firsthand what it feels like to watch someone you love make choices that could kill them.

While drugs, alcohol, and nicotine are addictions we can easily identify and define as clearly unhealthy, the fact is what many of us are doing to our bodies with the food we eat and the way we eat is equally dangerous. Not unlike the disregard that alcoholics and drug addicts have for their bodies, we abuse our bodies with yo-yo dieting, with weight-cycling, and with highly processed, high-fat, high-sugar, and high-chemical foods. We wash everything down with excessive caffeine, energy drinks, and sodas.

Continuously dieting is an abuse of our body. We're either following some kind of a restrictive diet, succeeding or failing on that diet, or starting yet another new fail-proof weight-loss plan.

If we're "succeeding on a diet," chances are we'll reward ourselves at some point (over the next few hours or days) with "just a bite" of a forbidden food—a bite that will most likely lead to another—and another. If we're "failing on a diet," we'll punish ourselves with harsh words of judgment ("I'm such a fat failure. Why do I bother trying?") followed by a bowl (box?) of sugary cereal or maybe a bowl (bag?) of salty potato chips. And if we're about to start a new diet, we'll most likely have a private going-away party/binge, featuring any number of the foods we're about to brutally deprive ourselves of, a swan song sandwich, or a farewell order of fries.

Remember, diets don't work.

Changing the habits we have concerning our relationships with food will involve commitment and discipline. But it's a one-day-at-a-time discipline that will last for the rest of our lives. This isn't a temporary six-week program, a one-week liquid fast, a 1200-calorie-a-day regimen, or a carbohydrate-restricted menu.

Living life to the fullest every day and treating our bodies with respect and love is a far more attainable goal than any of the destructive and often worthless diet programs that we've repeatedly subjected ourselves to. Success in every area of life is really about putting God first and allowing everything else to follow in a natural progression. And with regards to food, there's nothing more natural than eating. We've just distorted it by trying to control it for all the wrong reasons.

Perhaps another one of the reasons we've become the fattest nation on earth is because we've lost sight of the original intention of food. Food is intended to nourish us so we can be in the best possible condition to worship God and do His will. It was never intended to be the object of our affection—to become the substance we essentially worship.

For many of us, food represents far more than what God intended for it to be.

We all have the ability to affect the quality of our lives, and God has given us a responsibility—a mandate—to take care of ourselves, and in some instances to take care of others as well.

Nutritional Gatekeepers

A gatekeeper is a person who controls access to something, such as an entrance to a building, park, or secured area. Today, the term is often used metaphorically to refer to individuals who decide whether a message will be distributed. For example, a news editor decides which stories to print, a doorman who to allow in, or a business manager who is permitted access to his client. Gatekeepers have a responsibility to protect that which is under their care. Ideally, they have wisdom and discernment as they fulfill this responsibility. In many instances gatekeepers also have a great deal of power and control.

There is a powerful gatekeeper in every home today—the person who is responsible for buying, preparing, providing, and serving the food that is eaten in the home. Let's take that a step further. A nutritional gatekeeper is also responsible for the health and well-being of those they are feeding. Those of us who are gatekeepers of our family's health and nutrition must become more aware of the food we are buying and preparing for our children. Of equal importance is educating our children for the time when they are on their own and will need to make choices based on what they have learned from us.

I recently took someone grocery shopping who only had $26 to spend on food for two weeks. I encouraged him to look at ways to stretch those dollars to get the most nutritional bang for his buck by purchasing eggs, milk, chicken, and other basic staples, but instead he chose to buy nine frozen pizzas.

Where exactly do our kids first learn about food and nutrition? From the nutritional gatekeepers in their homes.

> You are the light of the world—like a city on a hilltop that cannot be hidden. No one lights a lamp and then puts it under a basket. Instead, a lamp is placed on a stand, where it gives light to everyone in the house. In the same way, let your good deeds shine out for all to see, so that everyone will praise your heavenly Father (Matthew 5:14-16).

Eat More Often

Many people try to eat less as stress levels climb. Yet going hungry can itself be very stressful, and feeding the body infrequently creates the alarm state that encourages fat storage. The solution: Eat more. I don't mean donuts and lattes, though. I mean low-calorie green food that you eat throughout the entire day. Adding foods with lots of antioxidants, water, fiber, and other nutrients can calm you and help your body relax.[1]

Health Food = Healthy Food

Women have been bombarded for years with images of how we're supposed to look. We've been programmed to believe that the measurement of our success is directly related to the measurements of our bodies. And it's no longer just women who are targeted with these unreasonable expectations—men have now become fair game as well. After all, how successful can you be if you don't have six-pack abs?

Health is one of the largest areas of concern for most Americans today. From books to videos, diets to fitness plans, and energy bars to supplements, people in our society are constantly searching for the newest ideas and interventions to improve or maintain their health. One of those relatively new ideas is a field of professional study where individuals guide and coach others with natural health questions from a biblical perspective. One such person is Joanna B. Faillace.

Joanna is a woman on a mission. She is a Certified Biblical Health Coach, author, and television host of the *Super-Naturally Healthy Cooking Show*. A while back Joanna and I participated on the speaker team for a special Thelma Wells *Ready to Win Conference* on a cruise ship to the Grand Caymans. One of Joanna's onboard presentations consisted of making her famous supernaturally healthy smoothies and I've been a fan ever since (of Joanna and her smoothies!).

She is also the nutritional gatekeeper for her husband and children. It was the realization of her responsibility to her family and their health that set her on a course that would change their lives and ultimately her own as well.

With a passion to educate, empower, and equip us with the tools we need to make healthy and godly choices in addressing our nutritional needs, I asked Joanna to share her story and tell us what we can do now to get supernaturally healthy.

> A few years ago God began revealing to me that I was being deceived by the advertising media with respect to my family's nutritional needs. My family was far from healthy—and as the nutritional gatekeeper I was greatly responsible for their poor nutrition. When God showed me the food I was buying (especially snack foods) was actually threatening my family's health, I realized this was no game! I was convinced I needed to change and began to pray, asking the Lord's forgiveness.
>
> I poured out my heart to Him and cried, "Lord, please forgive me. Tell me what I can do. I desire to be obedient to Your Word. By the power of Your Holy Spirit, give me the

knowledge, wisdom, and the self-discipline I need to make healthy food choices that will help restore and protect my family's health."

After that prayer, the Holy Spirit revealed a passage of Scripture that, somehow, I had missed in my 15 years of Bible study: "Don't you know that you yourselves are God's temple and that God's Spirit dwells in your midst?" (1 Corinthians 3:16 NIV).

Wow, talk about an eye-opener! That one verse dramatically changed my whole perspective on how I approached feeding my family. The Lord was revealing to me that I needed to make major changes—supernaturally healthy changes— in my family's diet or our health would soon begin to suffer drastically. What we eat is directly related to how we feel, think, act, and sleep. We desperately need to get back to eating the whole, supernaturally healthy foods that God created.

There are so many different types of foods on the market today that are missing vital nutrients, probiotics, antioxidants, and enzymes, which are the essential components of supernatural health. The scary truth is that junk foods are void of any significant nutritional value—they aren't really "food" at all— and in many cases their artificial ingredients can deplete our body's immune system, thereby setting us up as prime candidates for inflammation and diseases such as cancer, diabetes, obesity, and heart disease.

Think about it simplistically; if we eat junk, we will feel like junk. We can't put junk into our bodies and then expect to feel like a million bucks. The Bible says that "we reap what we sow," but it's also true that we reap what we swallow.

Don't play the devil's game! Don't be deceived by the world and Satan's lies because the truth is that these foods are actually "highly processed," meaning that they are loaded with artificial flavors, colors, sweeteners, toxic dyes, chemical preservatives like MSG, and incredibly high levels of sodium. My rule of thumb is that you know you're in trouble when you can't even begin to pronounce the ingredients.

I believe we can win the war against stress, fatigue, obesity, and disease. If we proactively fight back with God's whole super foods, natural herbs, and supplements, we can stop and in some cases even reverse the damage we've done. It's never too late to take that first step towards supernatural health and wellness.

It never ceases to amaze me that we take better care of our automobiles than we do our bodies. And surely our bodies—our temples of God—deserve regular tune-ups as much as our vehicles! We also deserve to be putting some high octane fuel into our tanks, and God's filling station can't be beat! Not only did He create whole and delicious foods for supernatural health and wellness, but also foods that can calm our anxious spirits in times of stress overload.

If you're craving something creamy, settle your spirit with a cup of organic, whole milk yogurt with fresh berries to fight the stress hormone cortisol. Or savor a few tablespoons of freshly made guacamole loaded with B vitamins, which stress quickly depletes. Broccoli, spinach, and zucchini are filled with fabulous, fat-flushing fiber. Fresh herbs are fragrant and flavorful, but did you know they also pack a punch of powerful antioxidants? For example, fresh rosemary contains antioxidants that help to fight free radicals and breast cancer. Rosemary contains Vitamin A and C to help prevent cataracts and infections and also provides energy and memory enhancement. You can also heat things up with thermogenic spices like cayenne, ginger, mustard, parsley, anise, bay, and cinnamon, which stimulate metabolism, improve glucose levels, and remove water weight. For those battling cancer, there is some very encouraging news. Berries are packed with lots of fiber and contain a powerful organic compound called ellagic acid, which in several studies has been shown to target and destroy cancer cells. Healthcare professionals have been telling us for years that we need to drink lots of water, but that means pure water, not water that contains caffeine or diet soda or chemicals.

In addition to eating healthy foods, try to exercise for thirty minutes per day at least five times per week. It's also extremely beneficial to get at least seven or eight hours of uninterrupted sleep each night. Insomnia seems to be an increasing issue in our society today, and that could be because of all the sugar, caffeine, and highly processed foods we are pumping into our bodies at alarming rates.

Last but not least, one of the most important supernaturally healthy things we can do in our lives is to begin and end our days in prayer. I believe that prayer is the key to inner peace because it is our direct line of communication with God. Spending quiet time with Him every day is the best supernaturally healthy method to calm our restless hearts and bring peace to our spirit.

The first edition of *Joanna's Super-Naturally Healthy Families Cookbook* is available now at her website, along with tons of valuable information for how you can begin an entirely new lifestyle filled with health, vitality, and God's very best. You can visit her website at supernaturallyhealthy.net.

Fast Food

Joanna touched briefly on an aspect of nutrition (and I use the word "nutrition" loosely) that has literally changed our entire culture. Today, fast food has become the most socially accepted addiction we've ever known. Unfortunately, the magnificent obsession we have with getting food as quickly as possible whenever and wherever we want it is taking its toll. For many of us, this magnificent obsession has little to do with enhancing the relationships around us, becoming instead the foremost relationship we enhance.

What have we lost as we've gained speed and convenience?

It seems there is also a systematic plan to encourage overeating. Cashiers in most fast food restaurants are now trained to ask customers if they want to supersize their order. In fact, "supersize" is now a word in Webster's dictionary. A major contributor to the obesity epidemic in the United States is an overdependence on fast food. We place our order, drive up to a window, hand over money, and get our drug-in-a-bag fix.

When did fast food become the acceptable opiate of the masses?

Fast food can be fatal food.

The Birth of Fast Food

As automobiles became more affordable following the First World War, drive-in restaurants became more and more popular. Walter Anderson built the first White Castle restaurant in Wichita, Kansas, in 1916, introducing the limited menu, high-volume, low-cost, high-speed hamburger restaurant. Among its innovations, the company allowed customers to see the food being prepared. White Castle was successful from its inception and spawned numerous competitors. We were hooked.

In 1940, Richard and Maurice McDonald opened the first McDonald's in San Bernardino, California. The two brothers became fast-food pioneers when they introduced the Speedee Service System in 1948 and began franchising their concept in 1953. In 1954, Ray Kroc, a milkshake machine salesman, partnered with the brothers. In 1961, he purchased the company from them for 2.7 million dollars.

Today, McDonald's sells about as many hamburgers in one day— 15 million—as it did in all of 1953. It's the world's largest chain of hamburger and fast-food restaurants, serving around 64 million customers every day.[61]

Hidden Truth—Hidden Harm

Then there's the ugly reality of where all of this fast food is coming from that's simply far too unattractive for most of us to address. How much do we really know about the food we eat at fast-food restaurants and all-you-can-eat buffets, or even the food we buy at our local supermarkets and serve to our families?

Food, Inc. is a documentary that lifts the veil on our nation's food industry, exposing how our nation's food supply is now controlled by a handful of corporations that often put profit ahead of consumer health, the livelihood of the American farmer, the safety of workers, and our own environment. *Food, Inc.* reveals surprising and often shocking truths about what we eat, how it's produced, and who we have become as a nation. The filmmaker takes his camera into slaughterhouses and factory farms where chickens grow too fast to walk properly, cows eat feed pumped with toxic chemicals, and illegal immigrants risk life and limb to bring these products to market at an affordable cost.

It was virtually impossible for me to eat a chicken nugget after I learned how they are made. I'm familiar with a chicken leg, a chicken breast, and chicken wings, but can you tell me what part of the chicken the nugget comes from? Think about it.

The Bottom Line

Knowledge is power, and that holds true especially when it comes to the food we are putting inside our bodies and inside the bodies of those we love and are called to protect.

Try buying only whole foods and cooking from scratch more often. Begin to pay more attention to reading food labels, especially when it comes to the sugar, fat, and artificial ingredients. Looking at the protein level is also critical—the higher the better. We need all the power possible as we change our eating habits and set healthy boundaries with food.

> And so, dear brothers and sisters, I plead with you to give your
> bodies to God because of all he has done for you. Let them be
> a living and holy sacrifice—the kind he will find acceptable.
> This is truly the way to worship him (Romans 12:1).

What to Do First

Stop dieting.
Stop eating unhealthy foods.
Stop feeding unhealthy foods to your family.

What to Do Next

Learn how to read food labels and what to look for.
Go hunting through your pantry and get rid of the bad stuff.
Make room for the good stuff and go grocery shopping.

Conduct a search-and-destroy food audit mission. Go through your refrigerator, cupboards, pantry, and anywhere else in your home where food lurks, and remove all junk food. Gather up ice cream, candies, frozen pot pies, chips, cookies, and especially those highly-processed snack foods that seemed a good idea at the time. Throw it all in the trash. Don't give this unhealthy food to someone else, no matter how much money you spent on it. Think of yourself as a drug addict. You desperately want to clean up your life but you're hesitant to destroy your existing stash of drugs because, after all, you spent a lot of money on those drugs. Might as well give them to someone else so the money won't be wasted, right?

Wrong.

Chapter 12

The Eating Experience

If we're serious about honoring God by taking care of the bodies He's given us, a significant boundary that needs to be set with food is how we experience the act of eating.

I once had a cartoon on my refrigerator that showed a harried looking woman standing in front of an open refrigerator eating directly from a bowl, with the optimistic (and false) caption, "Foods ingested while standing contain half the calories."

Another variation of that cartoon could be a picture of a mom driving a car or van with children buckled into their car seats and a caption that reads, "Foods ingested while driving 55 miles per hour contain fewer calories than those ingested sitting still."

Alas, neither of those scenarios are true, and may, in fact, be contributing factors to the increase in our weight and the decrease in our peace and sanity.

Have you ever parked alongside someone who is getting into or out of their vehicle with kids and the inside of their car or van looks like a scene from *Hoarders*? I can't possibly be the only person who has noticed this. Mom or Dad opens the door to assist children in or out, revealing a car filled with trash, beverage cups, food wrappers and bags, stained carpets, coloring books, pencils, markers, even articles of clothing like a stray shoe or sock.

This is wrong on so many levels. It isn't funny, and it's where many of us—including our precious children—are eating the majority of our meals today.

We've replaced a four-legged table with a four-wheeled vehicle.

A Disappearing Tradition

We've become a nation of people who don't have enough time and/
or income to eat healthy. For that matter, we don't have enough time to
actually sit down with our family to eat at all. Even when we eat healthy
food, it's most likely being consumed on the run, in vehicles, or often
late at night before going to sleep. Sadly, our physical health isn't the only
thing suffering. Our family relationships just aren't what they used to be.

In generations past, countless boys and girls learned the valuable essen-
tials of life, love, liberty, and the pursuit of happiness by regularly attending classes at Dinner Table University. This was a respected institution,
a place where life lessons were taught by revered and tenured professors
known as Dad and Mom. Sometimes Grandpa and Grandma played key
roles, and aunts, uncles, cousins, and assorted in-laws were often available full- or part-time as trusted teachers' aides. Together, these knowl-
edgeable and often tenacious teachers shared a wealth of wisdom and a
healthy dose of opinion that helped to feed the minds and hearts of the
young students who sat nearby.

It was a time when feeding the heart with love and the mind with
knowledge was every bit as important as feeding the body. Discussions
on religion, politics, and current events prompted both solidarity and
heated debate. Intellect was nurtured, emotional and social skills were
honed, and manners were taught. Building character, instilling ethics,
and imparting values were also on the curriculum. It was a priceless education, and for the most part attendance wasn't optional.

Today, this venerable institution of advanced learning and account-
ability has become one of the many fast-food fatalities nearing extinction
as busy schedules, misplaced priorities, and unhealthy boundaries have
taken precedence over relationships. For many Americans, sitting at the
dinner table as a family is something that occurs sporadically throughout
the year, typically on holidays or at events when family members are suddenly thrust together, such as at weddings or funerals.

Visitors from other countries often comment how different life is in
the USA when it comes to the celebration of food and eating. In many
countries the act of eating is an adventure—a frequent ceremony to be

savored, where relationships flourish amidst the preparation of and partaking in food—nutritious food—fresh food—*healthy* food.

Eat Together at the Table

When actress Maria Bello was growing up in Norristown, Pennsylvania, high-spirited conversation around the dinner table was just part of the household's soundtrack, as she recounted in a recent interview. "My mom is great about gathering people around food to share their stories. She has a way of talking directly to folks and helping them with their issues and problems. We congregate in the kitchen not only because it smells so good but because that's where you find the best conversation."[1]

One of my favorite television shows is *Blue Bloods*, a police drama set in the heart of New York City starring Tom Selleck as Police Commissioner Frank Reagan. The program revolves around multiple generations of the Reagan family. Along with the requisite drama, chaos, and crisis resolution, every episode includes some type of family relationship issue and culminates with their long-standing tradition of eating together every Sunday night at the family home Frank now shares with Henry Reagan, his father. With sons, daughters, brothers, sisters, in-laws, and grandkids, there are usually ten to twelve people in attendance, ranging in age from eight to eighty. None of the food being consumed comes from a paper bag or tub. Nothing has been wrapped in paper or foil, or contained in a cardboard sleeve or box. Nothing includes corporate brand advertising. There's nary a logo in sight. In the fictional Reagan household, Dinner Table University is alive and well.

Yes, it's television, and yes, it's a fictional family. Yet there was a time when this tradition thrived, when relationships were seen as the star performers in life and food played the supporting role. Today, it's food—not family—that seems to be the glue that is holding our fractured hearts and souls together, but it's not doing a very good job of adhesion.

Ask God to reveal to you if eating together as a family at the dinner table is something that needs to occur more often in your home.

Feeding Future Leaders

It's estimated that children in America see approximately 10,000 food advertisements each year. When shown pictures, children were more likely to recognize Ronald McDonald or Wendy than the President of the United States. Even sadder, people on the street could recite the familiar slogan for a fast-food hamburger chain but not the Pledge of Allegiance.

School kids are the consumers of the present and the future. Knowing this, major corporations see profits soar by capturing that market for their products. The health of the purchaser takes a backseat to the health of the corporation's profits.

Today, many kids think of French fries as a vegetable, that Pepsi or Coke fulfills their needs for water, and that protein is best found in a quarter-pounder. Clearly, nutrition education is needed for parents to pass on to their children. We've become a nation where toxic food is acceptable and an environment of physical inactivity is normal. A country where cheap, fat-laden foods are easy to acquire. With the ever-popular Dollar Menu, you can feed a family of three for under ten bucks, including a burger, fries, and beverage for everyone. If you do the math, there's no comparison in what it would take to buy all of the fresh ingredients to prepare the same meal. Plus, there's the consideration of time—we're just too busy to shop, prepare, cook, and serve healthy food.

Sadly, it's not only easier but acceptable to fill our bodies and the bodies of those we are responsible for with unhealthy food.

The Pageantry of Excess

One of the first introductions many American children have to eating outside their home is via what I call the MGM version of dining. Larger than life and filled with every imaginable grandiose scenario, I'm talking about our magnificent obsession with all-you-can-eat buffet restaurants.

Today, kids grow up seeing food displayed in organized stations where it is elaborately presented in massive quantities in large, shell-shaped bowls or on glistening Lucite trays, on beds of lettuce, crushed ice, or on chopping blocks where overhead heat lamps shine down. A white-smocked chef cuts individual slices with a gleaming carving knife. Adorned with attractive garnishes of flowers, vegetables, or fruit, some buffets even have ice sculptures.

It's all very visual, and young people are growing up thinking this is how life is. What began as a popular method for feeding a large number of people with minimal staff has turned into a national pastime with frightening consequences.

Americans have taken this boundary-free dining style to a new level. The epitome of conspicuous consumption, nothing says indulgence like an all-you-can-eat buffet, where plates—and often waistlines—are overflowing, where food is delicious and available in copious amounts whenever we choose. Even better, we can see we're not alone. Everywhere we look there is tangible evidence that others share our magnificent obsession with food. The clamor around these modern-day feeding troughs at mealtime is a sight to see.

Seriously, who needs this much food? As you strive to set boundaries with food, my advice is to stay away entirely from fast food and all-you-can-eat buffet restaurants.

No Time for Health

Ever said something like this? "Even though I only work part-time, there aren't enough hours in the day to get everything accomplished. I'm just too busy driving the kids to their events, taking care of the house, taking care of my husband, and doing everything else I have to do. Even *thinking* about grocery shopping, preparing food, cooking food, and serving food is too much! It's easier and more affordable just to grab food from any one of a dozen fast-food restaurants near our house, or pick up a pizza on the way home."

If this sounds familiar—if this is something you often find yourself saying—then consider asking God to help you implement the necessary changes you must make as the nutritional gatekeeper in your family. Ask Him to give you insight about spending quality time at the dinner table with your family.

While setting boundaries with food is about learning how to stop using food as a substance to avoid painful emotions or difficult situations or circumstances, it's also, in part, about enhancing the overall eating experience while putting food in its proper place of priority in our lives. What follows are just a few of the reasons that we may be experiencing challenges not only with our weight, but in finding energy, vitality, or any kind of true quality of life.

1. We're eating high-calorie, high-fat foods throughout the day and late at night before going to sleep.

2. We're eating fast food in our cars and paying little attention to the actual act of eating.

3. We're eating so fast we don't even remember what we've eaten.

4. We're eating far too much food at a time. Our portions are out of control.

5. We're eating too much highly processed artificial food that doesn't supply our bodies with the nutrients they need to function properly. Chances are our internal engines haven't been operating properly in years.

6. We're eating an overabundance of food high in sugar and fat that alters our brain chemistry, acting like drugs, putting us on a roller coaster of highs and lows that short-circuit our actual appetite triggers and contribute to mercurial emotional mood swings.

7. We're consistently depriving ourselves of food we want, often triggering a binge on that very food during a weak moment.

This list could continue for several pages. Does anything here ring a bell in your life? If so, write about it in your journal. Ask God to reveal the specific items He wants you to address, and how to take steps to address them when you develop your written plan of action in a later chapter.

A Healthy Way to Eat

Weight loss surgery forced me to adopt healthy habits for eating that I was unable to adopt on my own—habits everyone could benefit from. These are healthy habits that can reduce our weight, help us maintain a healthy weight, and restore our energy and vitality. Most importantly, they are habits that can help us separate food from our emotions, forcing us to listen to what our hunger is really telling us.

1. Eat slowly and chew your food.

2. Obtain the majority of your calories from protein.

3. Fill up on protein first, not on empty calories or high-fat, high-carb calories.

4. Limit sugar.

5. Limit carbohydrates.

6. Do not eat anything in your car.

7. Do not buy or eat fast food, fried food, processed foods, or artificial foods.

8. Eat when you're hungry and stop when you're full.

9. Listen to what hunger is, and listen to what full is.

10. Read food labels and know what to look for and stay away from.

11. Eat several small meals throughout the day. Portion control is critical.

12. Take a multivitamin with iron.

13. Get frequent medical checkups, including periodic blood tests.

14. Weigh yourself often to stay aware, not to punish or reward yourself.

15. When clothes are too big, get rid of them.

16. Do other meaningful things in your life so food and eating aren't the only source of enjoyment you have.

How Can We Tell What Processed Food Is?

Start by reading the label. If it has ingredients you can't even pronounce and wouldn't recognize if they stared you in the face, it's probably processed. If it's in cardboard, aluminum, or a vacuum-sealed pouch, chances are it's a highly processed food. If it has a shelf life to infinity and beyond, it's probably processed.

It's an irrefutable fact that if we eat less and exercise more we will lose weight. But eating less doesn't mean starving yourself for a few days and then binging. Eating less doesn't mean living only on salad and depriving yourself of protein and other necessary vitamins and minerals. Eating less doesn't mean only when others see you eat. The eating less I'm referring to is all about portion control. You can eat whatever you wish, just less of it. Hopefully, "whatever you wish" will soon consist primarily of nutritional, healthy foods that honor and respect your body.

Chapter 13

Dreams and Goals

It hasn't been surprising to me that many of the caring moms and dads I meet or hear from in response to *Setting Boundaries with Your Adult Children* are also dealing with health- and weight-related issues. Those of us facing that situation spend so much time taking care of our adult kids within the dysfunctional relationships we've created that we neglect our own health, our own dreams, and our own goals.

It's often the same case when we've neglected to set healthy boundaries with difficult people in our lives such as employers, coworkers, siblings, spouses, or ex-spouses. So many of us live from day to day on emotional roller coasters, it's no wonder the comfort of food calls out to us throughout the daylight hours and often late into the evening.

It may not be an adult child or another person in our life that short-circuits our pursuit of our dreams, but many of us who have difficulty setting boundaries with food will also find ourselves roadblocked from pursuing our dreams and goals as effectively as possible.

Our time on this planet is limited, and a sad consequence in living with a lack of healthy boundaries is that we often end up with a life that has basically been put on hold, a life that's not being lived authentically. We've either been accepting responsibility for someone else's life (thus relegating our own to a lesser value), or we've been coasting on cruise control, just waiting for the right time to begin our lives.

Friends, the right time is right now.

It's time to seize the moment and live the lives God has called us to live. If we don't pay attention to our life's purpose, our calling, and achieving the dreams of our hearts, who will?

Three Life-Changing Questions

I ask three questions at the start of my SANITY Support workshops for struggling parents who are caught in the bondage of dysfunctional relationships with adult children. Most often, the response I get is a deer-in-the-headlights stare.

1. What would you do with your life if you weren't so wrapped up in the ongoing drama, chaos, and crisis that surrounds your life with your adult child—if you weren't dealing with the never-ending sagas of their unemployment, addictions, financial challenges, and poor choices?

2. What would you do with the time if you stopped being responsible for the consequences of their choices?

3. What would you do with the money if you stopped funding their lives and stopped trying to solve their problems with your checkbook?

By the time they seek SANITY Support, many of these precious souls have spent countless hours—and often countless dollars as well—trying to help their adult kids. In so doing, they've all but lost track of who they are as separate individuals—children of an almighty God.

But something amazing happens when we begin to set healthy boundaries in our lives, when we put God first, when we begin to say no to the roadblocks in our path, when we begin to understand what it means to walk in our own calling and purpose, and when we begin to find sanity, fully commit ourselves to God, and trust that He is in control. We begin to experience life.

> Trust in the LORD and do good;
> dwell in the land and enjoy safe pasture.
> Take delight in the LORD,
> and he will give you the desires of your heart.
> Commit your way to the LORD;
> trust in him and he will do this:
> He will make your righteous reward shine like the dawn,
> your vindication like the noonday sun (Psalm 37:3-6 NIV).

What Are *Your* Goals?

Where do you think your true calling is? Are you living in the truth and light of that calling? If not, why not? How many years have we wasted doing things we don't really want to do? Being people we don't want to be? Living lives we never imagined for ourselves? When was the last time you focused on your passion, your purpose, and God's plan for your life?

When losing weight (and keeping it off) has been a consistently unaccomplished (or short-lived) goal for years—even decades—it's easy to see how discouraged and unmotivated we can be regarding setting goals in other areas in our lives. It's the same thing when we focus an unhealthy amount of time trying to help our adult children, or deal with challenging relationships with toxic relatives or difficult people.

We are so much more than the chaotic relationships we have, and oh so much more than what we weigh. We are children of a most awesome God who wants nothing more than to see us achieve all the dreams of our hearts—and then some! After all, He placed them there!

Often, we put things on hold. We'll get around to it later, we say, when we lose weight. Our weight has been the axis around which everything else in life spins.

I love to watch people discover (or rediscover) what it is they truly want to do with their own lives—outside of dealing with the challenging issues that have literally weighed them down.

I've been blessed over the past few years to work individually with people who yearn to tell their own stories, most often in the form of memoirs or autobiographies. Many of my fellow baby boomers long to process the years in ways that help them make sense of their journeys. Some wish to leave behind a legacy for their own children and grandchildren. In short, they want to know their lives counted.

Many of us who have experienced difficulty in setting boundaries now find ourselves at a place where we've forgotten what we wanted to do or be when we grew up—and now we're all grown up and find that something is missing.

But it doesn't have to stay that way. We can find that missing piece when we find peace. Today really can be the first day of the rest of our lives. We really can make choices to change.

In her book *Unlimited*, Jillian Michaels recalls a time when she wasted several years of her life pursuing a career as a Hollywood agent, a career she thought she wanted, but one in which every day she toiled away miserably. When she was fired she was initially devastated, but the situation forced her back into personal training, something she had done for years but had put on the back burner in favor of the new career. "Almost immediately I remembered the strength and joy I'd gotten out of being healthy and helping others do the same. I began to understand that my true calling was in the world of health and wellness."[1]

Let's explore what Jillian discovered.

Your Life Purpose

I spent many years building a career in nonprofit development and fundraising. I enjoyed the work and the challenges. Mostly, I enjoyed the writing—newsletters, proposals, press releases, and business plans. I'd also had some success as a freelance writer, with articles published in *Ladies' Home Journal, Cosmopolitan, Woman's World*, and *Shape* magazines. When I became a Christian I felt the call to write about my journey of faith, a calling that has increased year-after-year. It's been quite a road as I've partnered with some incredible publishers to actually see my writing dreams come true. Yet it hasn't been easy, as the author of *Listen to Your Hunger* attests.

> Achievement is hard. Eating is easy. Sometimes, eating recalls past achievement in early years and becomes a substitute for current accomplishment in the here and now.
>
> Listen to the hunger. What do you want to achieve? Do you want to go back to school and get a degree? Would you like to start your own business? Have you always wanted to learn to ski? Do you feel your present job is a dead end, and are you staying in it because that's easier than looking for a new one?
>
> When you think about taking action to fulfill one of your ambitions, do you get scared or discouraged and decide to have something to eat? All too often, an overeater will choose the immediate, short-term gratification of food instead of working toward a long-term goal.

Acknowledging our desires and dreams is the first step toward realizing them. Sit down and take time to think about three specific goals you want to accomplish by this time next year. Write them down on paper. For example,

1. a more interesting job
2. a better relationship with a family member
3. a firmer body
4. improved self-esteem[2]

What's Your Dream?

In her book *Girl Perfect: Confessions of a Former Runway Model,* Jennifer Strickland recounts her journey from the fashion world to God's Word. As a Ford model she was named the Face of the 90s, and has worked around the globe, most notably for Giorgio Armani on the runways of Milan. At 17, Jennifer was offered a modeling contract from world-renowned agent Nina Blanchard and an academic scholarship to the University of Southern California.

A week after her high school graduation she was on her own in Hamburg, Germany. Following her modeling dreams, Jennifer's college years were a whirlwind living in Europe in the summer, working in Germany, Paris, Greece, Australia, and Milan, and then coming back to Los Angeles for school in the fall. She juggled TV commercials, ad campaigns, catalogs, and classes. She grew up fast. However, Jennifer discovered that she lived in an imperfect world based on the myth of perfection. In order to make it as a model, she learned to wear masks.

Jennifer's story is an honest, authentic look at a world where so many young women are, quite literally, starving for love. A world where illusion replaces reality and little-girl dreams give way to painful, frightening nightmares.

It was during a time when she was down to mere skin and bones, using drugs, contemplating suicide, riddled with confusion, and haunted by loneliness that she discovered a perfect love that filled the emptiness in her heart. That was when she discovered the danger of pursuing a dream without God's blessing.

Today, as the Founder of Jennifer Strickland Ministries, she shares the principles of true beauty, leading girls and women to the lasting knowledge of who we are in God's sight: His beloved daughters, mothers, wives, sisters, and friends, handcrafted to reflect His glory to the world.

> Do you have a perfect dream for your life? It may not be your father's, your mother's, your sister's or your brother's dream for you. But that's all right…What matters is what God's dreams are for your life. What does he want to "work out" in you?… What could his plans be? What are the blueprints he carved out just for *you*? Ask him. Say to him, what is your perfect dream for me, God? Show me! Work it out for me! He loves prayers like that. They are invitations for him to show his power, his strength, and his love for you!
>
> You can begin discovering God's perfect dream for you by looking at your gifts and talents. What are you good at? Certainly we know we are much *more* than meets the eye. Psalm 139:13 says God formed our "inward parts." He formed our flesh, but also he formed our souls. What ignites passion in you? What do you care about? What makes you feel beautiful and worthy, like you are contributing to the earth? It is the answers to these questions that can lead you to the purpose God had for your life when he first formed you.[3]

Without censoring yourself, write down the dreams you have and ask God to point you toward the places where He wants you to fulfill His purpose and glorify His name. Ask Him to reveal the dreams He has for your life and to open doors to help make them come true.

Chapter 14

Making the Choice to Change

Even though some of us have been caught up in the dance of dieting dysfunction for years, it's not too late to change if we want to. It's our choice to be conquerors, to claim what is written in Romans 8:37 (NIV), "In all these things we are more than conquerors through him who loved us."

In his book *Dealing with the CrazyMakers in Your Life*, Dr. David Hawkins sums this up artfully:

> You and I must be able to make choices freely. Unfortunately, if you have been struggling with crazy-makers in your life, you may be addicted—in a loose sense of the word—to these people. You may be obsessively bound up in trying to change them instead of focusing your heart and soul on loving God, letting Him change you, and giving you wisdom for better ways of dealing with the situation.[1]

I've often said, "The choices we make can change the story of our life." After reading literally thousands (and editing hundreds) of true short stories over the years for my *God Allows U-turns* anthologies there's no doubt in my mind that God is showing up and providing miraculous blessings in the lives of His children.

But it's a two-way street. God isn't sitting looking for people to randomly bless. It doesn't work that way. That's not to say He couldn't arbitrarily make the choice to bless anyone He chooses—after all, He is God.

But the fact is, He wants us to be invested in our journey. He wants to know we want to change as much as He wants to help us change. He has no desire to enable us. When we're ready to roll up our sleeves and do the work, make the choice to change, and follow God's blueprints for living, there's no end to what He can help us build.

Getting Unstuck

A while back I was stuck in a situation with two difficult people that all but paralyzed me. I agonized, lamented, whined, and complained to my inner circle of friends and advisers. We discussed my options, the consequences, and the increasing damage the situation was doing to my business, finances, health, and overall well-being. Things needed to change but I was stuck on the gerbil wheel—going around and around with no end in sight. In his book *Getting Unstuck*, Dr. Sidney Simon summed up what I was feeling:

> All the ways you can get stuck have one element in common. Change is required—but you can't seem to make change happen. Whether you want to stop biting your nails or whether you have endured a decade of abuse from a spouse or parent, *when you are stuck your ability to do anything about your situation seems to disappear.* Nothing seems able to get you moving, not your desire to be better, not your treasured goals and aspirations, not even the pain you feel. Threats, bribes, and impassioned pleas are not enough to move you.[2]

There was no doubt I was stuck and needed to move, but for the longest time I existed in a place of utter frustration and fear, unable to effectively articulate my needs and unable to promote effective change.

But in spite of the increasing oppression, something miraculous was happening as well. I was growing spiritually in ways I could never have imagined. I prayed like never before and refused to let Satan win the battle. Determined to stay the course I grew increasingly dependent on God's Word and His will to see me through. At the end of my rope and hanging on for dear life, I consistently sought wisdom and discernment from the Lord and from the wise individuals He graciously placed in my life for such a time as this.

As those closest to me watched things unfold, they offered prayer, support, unconditional love, and insight into Scripture that proved invaluable. Eventually, when I felt the Spirit of God telling me it was time, I found the strength to move from a state of insane inertia into a season of action and sanity.

There was a time I would have sought comfort and solace in recreational drugs, empty relationships, or most often in copious amounts of high-fat food to get through a painful season in life. I won't lie: There were countless times during this lengthy period of ongoing crisis when I wanted to drive to the grocery store specifically for potato chips, fried onion rings, and butter pecan ice cream—the trifecta of comfort foods that now, post-surgery, make me deathly sick. And I can't tell you how many times I stood in front of my refrigerator late at night, crying, the glow of the light casting a shadow on the dark kitchen, and wishing I had something to eat that would magically make everything better, even if only temporarily.

Although the destructive habit to automatically mask my true emotions by stuffing them down with food was long gone, the fact I was even considering it made me remember how fragile we can be during times of trial. How easy it can be to slip back into old negative habits if new positive habits haven't replaced them!

Throughout this difficult situation, God was doing powerful things in my heart, soul, and spirit as I sought wisdom and direction in His Word, and as He revealed truth to my heart.

When the time came to set firm and healthy boundaries in this situation, I was ready to change, guard my heart, and accept the consequences—and I had faith that Jesus could change the circumstances of my life.

> Guard your heart above all else, for it determines the course of your life (Proverbs 4:23).

When We Reach the End of the Rope

Scripture tells us of a woman who had reached the end of her rope, yet she still had faith that Jesus could heal her—that Jesus could change the circumstances of her life.

> As Jesus was on his way, the crowds almost crushed him. And a woman was there who had been subject to bleeding for twelve years, but no one could heal her. She came up behind him and touched the edge of his cloak, and immediately her bleeding stopped. "Who touched me?" Jesus asked. When they all denied it, Peter said, "Master, the people are crowding and pressing against you." But Jesus said, "Someone touched me; I know that power has gone out from me." Then the woman, seeing that she could not go unnoticed, came trembling and fell at his feet. In the presence of all the people, she told why she had touched him and how she had been instantly healed. Then he said to her, "Daughter, your faith has healed you. Go in peace" (Luke 8:43-47 NIV).

There's nothing saying we have to wait until we've reached the end of our rope to cry out, asking God to heal us. If you're ready to make changes in your life, you'll appreciate some more insight from *Getting Unstuck*:

> I have a pleasant surprise for you. Nowhere is it written that you must suffer terribly before you change. In many instances you need not suffer at all, and you certainly do not have to endure prolonged pain, frustration, or uncertainty.
>
> Hitting bottom is what *you* make it. The bottom does not have to be the gutter or the coronary care unit. It need not be a welfare line or a psychiatric ward. Bottom is the place and the moment *you* decide you want to be happier, healthier, more creative, successful, or fulfilled than you already are. When you want to get unstuck and move forward, you have to hit your own bottom line and be prepared to rise above it. You can choose to *choose* to change, and you can begin *whenever* you please.[3]

Dr. Laura Schlessinger devotes many of her books and on-air radio time to people who make poor choices, people who are caught up in the bubble of insanity, "repeating the same behavior and expecting different results." This is particularly true when people have experienced an early childhood trauma. In her book *Bad Childhood, Good Life: How to Blossom and Thrive in Spite of an Unhappy Childhood*, she writes,

While there has been a whole cottage industry dedicated to those who believe and identify themselves as injured or handicapped by their childhoods—commonly known as victim, survivor, adult child of, or those with low self-esteem, or from a dysfunctional family—I believe that many people don't even realize that their childhood history has impacted their adult thought and behavioral patterns in unproductive ways. They don't realize that some of their less pleasant or destructive adult emotional reactions are reflexive responses forged by their unfortunate childhood challenges. They don't realize that much of their adult life has been dedicated to repeating ugly childhood dynamics in an attempt to repair deep childhood hurts and longings. They are reduced to believing that neither they nor life matters much anyway, not understanding that they have the power and the choice to make a good life.[4]

Sometimes we have to look away from our problems to let their solutions find us. Yet the question begs, How long do we allow ourselves to look away? A week? A month? Years, decades, a lifetime?

In her memoir *Then Again*, actress Diane Keaton shares that she looked away from her problems far too long as she fought a five-year battle with bulimia. In revealing this truth now she said, "I don't expect sympathy. I don't expect commiseration. I don't expect to be understood. What I expect is to be released from the burden of hiding."[5]

What are we hiding from?

Whatever it is, we can trust that it's no secret from God. When we're ready to make the choice to change, He will be right by our side. That said, the ball is entirely in our own court—and we've got to decide if we're going to show up and play the game.

The Eye of a Marksman

There are times when a Sunday sermon message hits the core of your heart—as though the pastor were an expert marksman, aiming effortlessly as he pierces the center of your being and leaves you profoundly changed. That's one of the reasons God calls us to be in community with other believers. He wants us to learn, grow, and change—and since the beginning of time He has called anointed men and women of God to share His word and His wisdom with us so we can do just that. Recently, I experienced one of those profound messages, a message for everyone struggling to find freedom from the bondage of insanity, from that place where our repeated behavior is getting zero results and we're finally ready to do what it takes to (gulp!) change.

Chuck Angel is the senior pastor at Harvest Church in Watauga, Texas. Pastor Chuck is not only a man after God's heart, but also a man after everyone's heart who walks through the doors of the rapidly growing church God has called him and his wife, Jill, to shepherd. He is passionate about connecting us with Jesus and about making the truth of Scripture come alive. He wants every heart to know God's love.

Pastor Chuck's message on change featured five key points. It was so powerful and so appropriate to those of us desiring to set healthy boundaries that I asked Pastor Chuck's permission to share those five critical components with you here.

What We Need to Be Intentional in Making Changes: The Five Change Constants

1. We need to be fully aware that things need to change.

It takes two things for this to happen. First, wake up and be self-aware. Second, have the courage to identify your need to change.

THE FIVE CHANGE CONSTANTS

1. We need to be fully aware that things need to change.

2. We need to turn to Jesus for help in changing.

3. We need to get in position for God to do great work in our life.

4. We need to be in partnership with God for the full release of His power.

5. We need to stay the course. Deep change has to be walked out.

Pastor Chuck has a witty sense of humor and always finds very obscure anecdotes to thread into his sermons. This was no exception. To illustrate the insanity of repeating the same behavior or habit and expecting different results, he said that in the cavalry there was a familiar saying: "When you're riding a dead horse, it's best to dismount." He went on to say that we need to be fully aware that things need to change. Whatever got us to this point probably won't get you to a new point, he said.

In other words, you have to change in order to change.

2. We need to turn to Jesus for help in changing.

Jesus Christ doesn't change but He is the authority for all change.

> I am the LORD, and I do not change. That is why you descendants of Jacob are not already destroyed (Malachi 3:6).

The bleeding woman grabbed the hem on the robe of Christ and was immediately healed. In her heart she believed and had faith that Jesus could save her and change her. "In our heart, where is our dependency for change?" Pastor Chuck asked.

3. We need to get in position for God to do great work in our life.

The bleeding woman humbled herself and went out to meet Jesus. "Our need can humble us or make us prideful," Pastor Chuck said. "We need to get over ourselves."

> In the same way, you younger men must accept the authority of the elders. And all of you, serve each other in humility, for "God opposes the proud but favors the humble." So humble yourselves under the mighty power of God, and at the right time he will lift you up in honor (1 Peter 5:5-6).

4. We need to partner with God for the full release of His power.

God can do anything He wants on His own without us. He doesn't need us, but He wants to be in relationship with us.

> For God is working in you, giving you the desire and the power to do what pleases him (Philippians 2:13).

Pastor Chuck reminds us, "If you want to see change you've got to do your part and He will do His part…Humble yourself and pray—that's your part. Pray and have faith that God will always do what He says He will do. We've got to do what God asks us to do, and if we show up, He will show up. Change is always about a partnership."

5. We need to stay the course. Deep change has to be walked out.

We need to press on and move forward—no matter how difficult the journey.

"Our sincerity may be real, but we've got to remain in the game through it all. Just look at what happened to Lot's wife," Pastor Chuck said. God "brought tremendous change to their family, but she couldn't stay on course, and looking back ended her life."

> No, dear brothers and sisters, I have not achieved it, but I focus on this one thing: Forgetting the past and looking forward to what lies ahead, I press on to reach the end of the race and receive the heavenly prize for which God, through Christ Jesus, is calling us (Philippians 3:13-14).

Be faithful and apply these Five Change Constants, and God will show up and change your life.

Ask God to Help

I hope you'll find Pastor Chuck's message of the Five Change Constants to be helpful as you navigate the terrain of change. The Bible is filled with stories of ordinary people who did extraordinary things with God's help. There is no doubt that He can do the same today for you.

You can choose to stop being whipped about by the winds of destructive habits and past choices. It's all about showing up, having faith, and trusting God to do what He promises He will do.

Chapter 15

Is Surgery the Solution?

Before we move to Part Two and the Six Steps to SANITY, I'd like to address the hot-button topic of weight loss surgery. If you're considering weight loss surgery (WLS,) please do not take lightly the important emotional and spiritual progression needed in preparing for this life-changing procedure. WLS gave me many tools to help me become *physically* free of the bondage to food, but it wasn't until I came to understand God's love for me and had His hope and trust for me firmly ensconced in my heart and soul that I was able to be *emotionally* free of the bondage to food.

Over the past few years I've watched fellow WLS brothers and sisters gain back weight because they never dealt with their emotional baggage before their surgery. Don't make that mistake. I was in a reasonably healthy emotional and spiritual place to take the major step—or at least in a far better place than I had ever been. A key in the success versus failure rate of this revolutionary and controversial surgery is our willingness to unpack the emotional baggage—to thoroughly clean the closets of our conscience and get rid of old thought patterns that no longer fit. We've got to be deliberate and intentional in choosing to change.

We all have defining moments in the layers of our lives: graduations, marriages, childbirth, the death of a loved one, medical emergencies—the list is endless. Although having weight loss surgery was indeed a defining moment in my life, it was the emotional and spiritual journey in the years before and after that really changed my life.

Before I could get the new body I have today I had to get a new head, and before I could get a new head I needed a new heart. I had to increase the love in my heart before I could maintain the surgically altered size of my stomach.

This was no easy task, as my heart was filled with decades of pain, anger, unforgiveness, shame, fear, and loss. Whether you are considering WLS or not, if you want to have long-lasting success in changing your relationship with food you'll need to do the same. You'll need to come to a place where your mind-body and head-heart issues can be truthfully identified and addressed—where substitution and avoidance no longer play a role. It won't always be easy, but if you are willing to try, I can assure you it will be an amazing journey.

The First Steps of the Journey

It took me years to reach the place where I was emotionally stable and spiritually strong enough to make an educated decision to undergo such a drastic weight loss procedure. The choice to have WLS should not be made quickly. I conducted a lot of research, and I prayed about it for a long time. I encourage you to do the same.

When I began to research WLS in earnest I had many questions. Who is a candidate for the surgery? Is there more than one type of WLS? If so, what are the differences? What exactly happens to the stomach in the surgery? How safe is it? Is it reversible? What is the success rate? Do people gain back their weight? What are the long-term nutritional consequences? Would my medical insurance cover it? Sometimes the questions seemed endless, and finding answers was tedious and frustrating.

Today, there is an extensive amount of information available online. In fact, the numerous resources at your fingertips now can become downright overwhelming. Since my surgery in October of 2000, when I had the *open roux en Y* gastric bypass procedure, there has been one particular WLS resource I've consistently turned to and often recommend: ObesityHelp.com. I'd encourage you to begin your research at this website, subscribe to their online publication, and participate in one of their many online support groups or chat rooms. They also have a magazine you'll want to subscribe to. OH Magazine and ObesityHelp.com have an established track record of professionalism, consistently remaining on the cutting edge of medical advances. Plus, they offer tools to track your weight, BMI, countdown clocks to surgery day, and more. Member profiles and before-and-after photos are encouraging and inspiring.

The Question of Faith

As I discussed this surgery with my faith-focused friends, one question seemed to be prevalent in most conversations: "Are we stepping outside God's divine plan by surgically altering the body He has given us?"

I'd answer by asking: Is it God's will to have surgery or chemotherapy if we have cancer, or have we stepped out of His divine plan by seeking help? Are we taking matters into our own hands by seeking aggressive treatment at the hands of a gifted physician? Is it God's will to surgically remove a bad appendix should it burst, or do we let nature take its course? Is it God's will to have a heart, lung, kidney, or liver transplant if it will keep us alive? Not such difficult questions if you believe that God has gifted surgeons and scientists with the abilities to diagnose illness and heal us when we're sick—and that for some of us being morbidly obese is indeed a sickness.

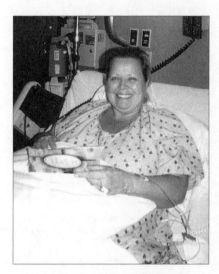

Day of surgery, October 10, 2000. Weight 280 pounds.

Alas, there are those within the faith community who do not see obesity as a physical disease, equating it instead as a weakness of will or lack of discipline. I believe well-meaning Christians are, in fact, doing great damage when they express negative comments regarding a surgical procedure that saves countless lives, and I ask such people to pray hard before admonishing anyone that it's not God's will to have weight loss surgery.

I don't believe those who are vocally against this procedure intend to be malicious or cause pain, but are instead misinformed, speaking only out of ignorance. This has happened before within the contemporary

Christian community when it comes to modern advances in medicine and nutrition.

Years ago it was unheard of in faith-based circles to discuss natural healing through the use of vitamins and herbal remedies. Anything concerning those topics was deemed "New Age" and quickly shunned. When I became a Christian this mindset was difficult for me to grasp. Vitamins and natural remedies had played an important part in my life for many years. I had spent almost two decades living in Southern California, a veritable Mecca of health-conscious hedonism. Throughout those years I had grown accustomed to taking vitamins and, whenever possible, using herbal remedies for health-related issues. I gave up a lot of bad habits when I became a Christian, and rightfully so, but it never occurred to me that alternative medicine was something sinful that I had to give up. So you can imagine my surprise when I asked a Christian bookstore owner for a book on natural healing! You'd have thought I was asking for a manual on Satan worship.

Today that is no longer the case, and one of the most comprehensive

DID YOU KNOW:

- The Surgeon General's *Report on Nutrition and Health* states that five of the ten leading causes of death in the United States are related to nutrition.

- Obesity is a major health problem affecting over six million people.

- Obesity is the second leading cause of preventable death in the United States. Tobacco is the first.

- Each year approximately 60,000 obese persons choose surgical methods (i.e., vertical banded gastroplasty and gastric bypass surgery) to permanently reduce their health risks. Most are more than 100 pounds overweight and have weight-related health problems.

books on the topic is now available in Christian and secular bookstores around the world. *Natural Health Remedies—An A-Z Family Guide* by Dr. Janet Maccaro, a brilliant and God-gifted nutritional expert, is a natural health book told from a decidedly Christian perspective. It has replaced my secular books on the topic and brings great insight and biblical truths about God's grand design for our bodies. I refer to it often for any number of health-related issues.

I had a host of weight-related health problems when I was first listed as morbidly obese on my medical chart, but it was another five years before I underwent the WLS procedure. The decision to have WLS isn't a vain cosmetic attempt to control our appearance, or an easy way out (this has been anything but easy). For many of us it's a vital, life-saving medical procedure; a tool that can help us to better help ourselves. And while I am a proponent of alternative medicine, after extensive research I also became a proponent of WLS for the morbidly obese patient. I had exhausted every means of traditional dieting for decades and my body was in danger. Weight loss surgery saved my life. Will it save yours or that of a loved one?

I thank God every day for giving the gift of healing to my surgeon's hands. I thank Him for giving me a second chance at living a life that does not revolve around weight-related illness. I am able to work more powerfully for the Lord today than ever before.

If you or someone you know is considering WLS, my best advice I can give is to pray, pray, and pray some more, and do your homework. In the meantime, I've included a list below you may find helpful.

- Keep a journal or diary. Begin the serious process of soul-searching. (Bravo, you've already begun this step here!)

- Research the types of WLS methods available and which is right for you.

- Meet with several bariatric surgeons to discuss their WLS methods and views.

- Learn about the lifelong vitamin and nutritional needs after WLS.

- Address life history issues that may be holding you back.

- See a licensed psychologist who specializes in weight-related issues.

- Attend several WLS after-care groups and listen to comments from WLS post-ops.

- Talk with your spouse and/or immediate family members. Ascertain their level of support.

- Decide which friends and family members you will tell about your impending WLS.

- Request pre-approval from your medical insurance company.

Head and Heart Health Comes First

I've heard countless objections over the years from people seeking WLS about the provision many health care providers mandate as part of their approval process for this surgery—a lengthy psychological evaluation and assessment. My insurance company required at least six private sessions over a minimum of six weeks with a licensed professional who specialized in WLS and who would attest—in writing—that I was indeed psychologically ready for the procedure.

I'll admit that at first I was miffed at the requirement. But it turned out to be unbelievably helpful, and I know the professional therapist I worked with had a great deal to do with that. She specialized in working with morbidly obese clients who were considering WLS, and she also had a great deal of experience in addressing the myriad issues surrounding violated boundaries.

It's important to do your homework with respect to the mental health care provider you are considering. Ask what their specialty is and find out how experienced they are. Attend WLS support group meetings and ask for personal references, call the bariatric surgeons in your area and ask who they recommend, conduct online searches, and don't be afraid to ask questions. As Christians, our faith is very important to us, and I always encourage fellow believers to make this aspect of counseling important as well. We are seeing more and more Christian counseling centers and services, and I encourage you to seek out these faithful professionals.

We are very keen on instant gratification—we want everything here and now. Yet the foundation of emotional balance must first be in place before we embark on WLS, and that takes time. For many of us, the building of that foundation will be even more life-changing than surgery. In school we must do our homework before we take the test. So, too, with WLS—before having surgery it is vital that we do our homework first. We have to get prepared.

I had done a great deal of damage to my body over the years with habitual weight cycling and destructive diets. I also had significant physical challenges after so many surgeries, with the prospect of more on the horizon soon if I didn't get my weight in check. Because of those components, I chose the additional tool that WLS provided me.

Yes, WLS changed my life, but the real, lasting change came when I opened my heart to hear God's call and relinquished everything to Him. The defining moment in my life came when I made a U-turn and allowed God to be in control of my life. God's love, peace, and joy filled that ever-present empty place in my heart.

Getting Ready for SANITY

Recently I watched one of my favorite movies, *P.S. I Love You*, a sweet love story based on the book by Cecilia Ahern about a young widow coming to terms with the death of her husband in a unique way. After a year of mourning she finally realizes, "Jerry is gone. I don't feel him here every minute of every day anymore." It's an epiphany that allows her to move forward in life—an epiphany that we need to experience in our relationship with food.

Food is the fuel our bodies need to live healthy and productive lives—it was never intended to control our lives every minute of every day. When we are constantly counting calories, carbohydrates, grams, points, or anything concerning our diet, we are focused on the food. When we're constantly mourning the foods we tell ourselves we can't have, or chastising ourselves for failing at yet another diet, we are focusing on the food.

Our goal is to stop focusing on food and start living our lives.

It was about a year after my weight loss surgery when I stopped consciously thinking about food. I remember it clearly. I was doing something

I had been unable to do when I was obese—gardening—when I realized my stomach felt empty and noticed that it was time for lunch. This is the natural progression for how our bodies have been designed—to eat when we're physically hungry and listen to the hunger. This was a liberating and emotional realization.

Therefore, from this day forward let's give ourselves permission to never go on a restrictive diet again, making the choices to live our lives the way God intends, with love, joy, peace, and SANITY.

It really can be as easy as that.

Part Two

SANITY
Makes a Comeback!

Chapter 16

The Power of SANITY

Establishing appropriate boundaries is essential to creating and maintaining mental, physical, emotional, and spiritual health. We've learned the value of looking at all the components that comprise a balanced life, and the importance of striving to address each of these areas in a deliberate and proactive way. We've discussed that for some of us, the violations to our boundaries have been severe, and gaining clarity and balance might require the additional help of a trained professional. For others, it might be enough to simply be aware of the emotional triggers that in the past sent us running to the refrigerator, pantry, or vending machine and learn to head them off at the pass by looking more closely at what we are avoiding by eating.

Whatever the driving issue that causes our boundary-setting challenges, the Six Steps to SANITY can be a powerful prescription to address the absence of boundaried living. The Six Steps can be the way we turn when we've been using food as a substitute to avoid painful and uncomfortable feelings—often rooted in our past.

Negative feelings don't go away just because they have no relevance to our lives today. They go away when we dig them up and expose their roots to the sunlight of truth. Only then will they shrivel up and die, no longer choking out the seeds of love and life that for so long have been struggling to grow. Only then can we begin to see the Light.

SANITY is a way back to God.

Sadly, many of us don't even realize how far we've wandered.

177

What Is SANITY?

SANITY is what we gain when we shift our priorities and stop focusing on dieting, food, and on our weight—when we stop focusing on the problems of others, and on the situations and circumstances of life, and begin to focus on changing our own attitudes and behaviors, starting with our hearts.

SANITY comes when we make the heartfelt commitment to stop using food as a way to avoid addressing our emotional pain or as a substitute to fulfilling our needs. It comes when we begin understanding how much God loves us, has a plan and purpose for us, and wants to meet our every need in ways that food never can.

SANITY is living in the peace that comes when we put our trust in God.

> So don't worry about these things, saying, "What will we eat? What will we drink? What will we wear?" These things dominate the thoughts of unbelievers, but your heavenly Father already knows all your needs (Matthew 6:31-32).

As God makes a difference in us, He will make a difference in how we view—and use—food. As God becomes the nourishment of our spirits and souls, our desires to nourish our bodies in healthy ways will follow.

The Purpose of SANITY

The goal of SANITY is to help us protect and nurture our hearts—the center of all the vital activities of body, soul, and spirit, the center of our personality, our character. Remember what King Solomon tells us in Proverbs 4:23 (NIV), "Above all else, guard your heart, for everything you do flows from it."

The New Testament teaches that no man or woman is safe apart from Jesus Christ because there is evil and treachery in the heart. It is the heart that is strengthened by God, and Jesus said that He came to "comfort the brokenhearted" (Isaiah 61:1). Our highest calling as Christians is that of being in relationship to Jesus. Only then can we begin to sort out how to live an obedient life in an immensely precarious, haphazard world. Only then can we make sense of the senseless and be able to see God at work always in all ways.

The need to set healthy boundaries in life often becomes clear to us when we're in the throes of crisis and trauma as a result of having weak or nonexistent boundaries in the first place. When, as though a curtain is lifted on the stage of our lives, we can see with painful clarity our woeful existence and our need to change. It's a revelation of the heart that opens our eyes, ushering in a profound season of change.

The Heart of SANITY

When the Spirit of God is awakened in our hearts and souls and we've reached the end of our self-directed, self-reliant, and self-centered lives, God can begin to show us that nothing is too hard for Him, no sin is too difficult for His love to overcome, and no failure is so great that He cannot make it a success.

The Six Steps to SANITY is about helping us replace old habits with new. However, without the character of Christ as our guide and the grace of God always in our sight, we can become slaves to the habit of trying to *break* habits. Oswald Chambers said,

> Habits are built up, not by theory, but by practice. The one great problem in spiritual life is whether we are going to put God's grace into practice. God won't do the mechanical; He created us to do that; but we can only do it while we draw on the mysterious realm of His divine grace. When we begin to work out what God has worked in, we are faced with the problem that this physical body, this mechanism, has been used by habit to obeying another rule called sin; when Jesus Christ delivers us from that rule, He does not give us a new body; He gives us power to break and then re-mould every habit formed while we were under the dominion of sin.[1]

When we realize the habits we've formed around food are indeed sinful, and Jesus Christ has delivered us from sin, it enables us to walk in a new light of understanding concerning what we're eating, how we're eating, and why we're eating, and to make changes that will last a lifetime and not just for the duration of another short-term deprivation diet.

THE SIX STEPS TO SANITY

S— *Stop* your own destructive patterns.

A— *Assemble* a support group.

N— *Nip* excuses in the bud.

I — *Implement* a plan, define your boundaries.

T— *Trust* the voice of the Spirit.

Y— *Yield* everything to God.

Chapter 17

S—Stop Your Own Destructive Patterns

The first step in the Six Steps to SANITY is to *stop*. It sounds rather simple, but for many of us caught up in the drama, chaos, and crisis of living in a world where unhealthy boundaries thrive, especially one in which food has taken on a life of its own, the idea that we can actually make the personal choice to stop the insanity is sometimes an amazing revelation.

Stopping ourselves from eating when we're not physically hungry, stopping our negative self-talk, and stopping any number of self-defeating habits must become deliberate choices we make in our lives. We've got to make a conscious effort to ask the Lord to help us break our destructive patterns of behavior.

After looking up "morbidly obese" in the dictionary when first confronted with the painful truth of my physical condition, I began conducting online searches for more information. This led to medical studies, books, blogs, reports, and more. It was a maze of information overload, but after a while there seemed to be a common thread emerging: boundaries.

By this time in my life I wasn't unfamiliar with the term. In processing the pain of my past in counseling over the years, I understood that the violation of my boundaries as a child, and again as a survivor of domestic violence, had left tire tracks of damage on my heart. However, I had never drilled any deeper into the actual study of boundaries or what the Bible said about boundaries.

When God began revealing to me that it was time to take a hard look at my lack of boundaries, I was ready for the task. I knew that my lack of boundaries had contributed not only to my obesity but also to the challenges I was still having with my adult son. Maintaining the status quo was no longer an option, and I began to see that before I could effectively move forward there were many things I had to *stop* doing. So I picked up my notebook and I wrote STOP at the top of the page. I began listing things that *I* thought God would most likely want me to stop.

Thankfully, God didn't allow me to spend too much time on this fruitless exercise before convicting me of what *He* really wanted me to stop first.

> I will instruct you and teach you in the way you should go; I
> will counsel you with my loving eye on you (Psalm 32:8 NIV).

There I was, making a list of things I thought God would want me to stop without so much as inviting Him to join me, or asking Him to direct me toward His truth. The first thing I really needed to stop was trying to think for God. I was trying to be in control of this entire process myself instead of allowing the Holy Spirit to impart truth in my heart to help me change. I needed to ask God to open my eyes and teach me in the way I should go, to show me what He wanted me to stop.

Developing the spiritual habit of asking and listening for God's direction is a vital discipline that will contribute to our finding and keeping SANITY. It's important to *stop* walking in our own will and our own direction, and instead ask God to lead us.

Attitude Defines Our Altitude

Just as a critical spirit projected outward can damage the hearts and souls of others, when projected inward it can have the same damaging effect. If you've ever heard, "Don't be so hard on yourself," you may have a problem with your self-image lining up with God's image of you.

When we have boundary issues with food there's a likelihood we have experienced cruel judgment and rejection at times in our lives, affecting our feelings of self-worth. When we have used food as a false boundary to protect ourselves, we may feel inadequate, fearful, and insecure. Our self-defeating statements are in direct opposition to what God sees.

I've heard it said that our "attitude defines our altitude." Even though

God's Word tells us in Isaiah 40:31 that we can "soar high on wings like eagles," if in our own hearts and minds we harbor negative thoughts and feelings of inadequacy, insecurity, or other self-defeating thoughts that diminish our true identity as children of Christ, we're going to be hard-pressed to see ourselves as God sees us. And it's critical in our journey to find SANITY that we learn to see ourselves through God's eyes.

The Bible teaches in 1 Samuel 16:7 that "The LORD does not look at the things people look at. People look at the outward appearance, but the LORD looks at the heart." Remember, SANITY is based on the premise that we must guard our hearts. Therefore, another critical step in finding SANITY is to stop our negative self-defeating self-talk.

Stopping Our Own Destructive Habits

While there are going to be many similarities in the things we have to stop when it comes to setting boundaries with food, such as our need to stop eating high-fat, high-sugar, and highly processed fake foods, there may also be things the Holy Spirit lays on our hearts to stop that we might not immediately associate with this issue—things we might not be aware of or don't think are important. Remember, God's ways are not our ways. He thinks differently than we do, and it's our responsibility to get on His page, not vice versa.

This first step is so important in finding SANITY that my friend Carole Lewis, the bestselling author of *The Divine Diet* and the director of First Place, wrote an entire book about it. Here's a sampling of what she has to say regarding "The Jolt that Moves Us."

> Stopping destructive thoughts and actions has the power to open up a life you think could never be possible. This good life, filled with meaning and purpose, is well within your grasp. To experience it, however, you must stop the bad on the way to starting the good.
>
> Can a changed life come about as simply as choosing to stop doing something and praying for God's help in the process? Absolutely. As we learn to "catch" our destructive thoughts when they come to mind, we can take captive those thoughts to make them obedient to Christ. When we adjust

destructive thoughts before they take root in our minds and hearts, we can change the destructive behaviors that result from those thoughts.[1]

Carole uses the following Scripture verse to further strengthen this point.

We destroy every proud obstacle that keeps people from knowing God. We capture their rebellious thoughts and teach them to obey Christ (2 Corinthians 10:5).

They say the first step in any journey of growth is often the hardest, but unless we take that crucial first step we'll never arrive at our destination. This first step can bring a level of illumination to our lives that will enable us to see more clearly than we have for years.

Remember the oft-quoted definition of insanity? *Insanity is repeating the same behavior and expecting different results.* It's time to *stop* repeating the destructive patterns that have not produced the desired results, and to step back to gain a better perspective on the situation.

Accomplishing these four "Stop Steps" can be life-changing.

1. *Stop* repeating our destructive patterns.

2. *Stop* ignoring our personal issues.

3. *Stop* being alone in our confusion and pain.

4. *Stop* pushing God out of the picture.

1. Stop Repeating Our Destructive Patterns

Talk is cheap.

It's one thing to say we want to set healthy boundaries with food, but it's another thing entirely to commit to change and doing the necessary work to embark on a journey that will transform our lives. Actually implementing the Six Steps to SANITY is a decision that should be made with a great deal of thought and prayer. We must be ready, willing, and able to give the process of change our total commitment, and we must be fully convinced of the need to stop repeating our destructive patterns, whatever they may be. We'll only stand strong if our initial commitment to stop is truly something we're ready to do and know that God is calling us to do.

In her book *The Emotionally Destructive Relationship*, Leslie Vernick addresses the truth about change, and how it begins when we stop.

> The most painful step in any healing process is often the first one. You must face the ugly truth that you're in a destructive relationship and that you are the one who has allowed it to continue. Just like a person wouldn't begin chemotherapy unless she first accepts that she has cancer, you will not take the steps necessary to grow, heal, or change if you are still in denial. As long as you minimize the truth about your problem, you cannot become strong enough to challenge or change anything. Wherever you are, it is important you realize that stopping the destructive dance starts with you.[2]

The change starts with us when we face the ugly truth that we're in destructive relationships with food—and dieting—and eating—and it's time to *stop*. Whether it's compulsive eating, overeating, binging, purging, or excessive dieting, when food is being used as a substitute to avoid something else it is destructive. Other destructive patterns can be:

- Negative thinking/feelings
- Responding emotionally
- Mistrusting God
- Perpetuating insanity

2. Stop Ignoring Our Personal Issues

Boundaries come in all shapes and sizes. They can be healthy or violated, intrusive or distant, or safe and loving.

When we grow up in a dysfunctional family, healthy boundaries can be like speaking a foreign language. We have no idea what's being said. By the time we reach adulthood, many of us have acquired reasonably acceptable coping mechanisms to get by. But is "getting by" all we aspire to do? Doesn't God want (and promise) so much more than that?

I spent decades just getting by, but it wasn't until I checked myself into a one-month treatment program years ago to sort out the mess I had made of my own life that I first began to see my negative behaviors and destructive patterns (especially the enabling component) for what they were. Are there personal issues you may need to acknowledge? Ask God to reveal what He wants you to address. Think about it. Pray about it. Whatever the trial, rest assured that God will not give you more than you can handle. This is not merely a Christian platitude—it is God's truth.

> Blessed is the one who perseveres under trial because, having stood the test, that person will receive the crown of life that the Lord has promised to those who love him (James 1:12 NIV).

3. Stop Being Alone in Our Confusion and Pain

It's important not to isolate yourself during this time of change, no matter what you may be dealing with. We were created to be in relationship with God the Father and with other brothers and sisters in Christ. Additionally, there is nothing to be ashamed of if you feel the need to talk with a professional counselor or psychologist to get your life back on track. In fact, it could be the best call you ever make.

> Again, truly I tell you that if two of you on earth agree about anything they ask for, it will be done for them by my Father in heaven. For where two or three gather in my name, there am I with them (Matthew 18:19-20 NIV).

4. Stop Pushing God Out of the Picture

It's not unusual to turn (or return) to our faith during times of trial and tribulation. God will often use the most painful experiences to teach us the most profound lessons. But God is so much more than a lifeguard who is standing by ready to rescue us when we're drowning.

God created us for a love relationship with Him. He wants to be involved in *every* area of our lives. Unfortunately, we often assign God to a limited place in our lives. What kind of love relationship is that?

> Hear, O Israel: The Lord our God, the Lord is one. Love the
> Lord your God with all your heart and with all your soul and
> with all your strength (Deuteronomy 6:4-5 niv).

To be loved by God is the highest relationship possible, the highest position in life. Our relationship to God (Father, Son, and Spirit) is the single most important aspect of our life. God wants us to love Him with our total being. He created us for that very purpose. If our relationship with Him is out of line, everything else related to knowing, doing, and experiencing God's will is going to be out of balance as well.

This was certainly the case when I was so entrenched in enabling my adult son, and during the years I was using food as a false boundary, and most recently in a challenging relationship with a family member. In all instances, the messier the situations got, the less one-on-one time I spent with God. Not because I didn't trust Him—that was never the case. It was because the increasing boundary-related problems I was having began to consume me, robbing me of peace, joy, time, sleep, and eventually my health. I was so weary I couldn't see straight.

Thankfully, through the loving kindness and prayers of close friends and by the power of the Holy Spirit as I cried out for freedom from the bondage, I was able to get back on track, restoring the most important relationship in my life.

When We Stop, the Healing Starts

The "S" step in SANITY will set the course for all of the steps that follow. Hopefully, once we finally own up to our destructive patterns for what they are and admit how damaging they've become, we won't be able to continue the same behavior expecting different results. God willing, we will feel deep conviction in our souls to make choices that will change our lives.

When we are finally ready to stop and say, "Lord, it's time for me to stop. I can't do this on my own any longer; I need Your help," God will often make Himself known in miraculous ways.

> Come to me, all of you who are weary and carry heavy bur-
> dens, and I will give you rest (Matthew 11:28).

As a reminder of the *STOP* measures you'll need to employ, photocopy this list and put it in a place where you'll see it often—the refrigerator door, bulletin board, bedroom mirror, or some other prominent place.

STEP 1 TO SANITY— STOP

THINGS TO STOP, STARTING NOW

Stop repeating the same responses and expecting different results.

Stop my own negative behavior and destructive patterns.

Stop ignoring my own personal issues.

Stop being alone in my pain.

Stop pretending things are going to be fine if I continue as I have been.

Stop putting off the changes that must be made.

Stop feeling guilty for past mistakes and choices.

Stop demanding that other people change.

Stop making excuses for the negative behavior and/or choices of others.

Stop engaging in arguments, debates, or negotiations—no verbal volleyball.

Chapter 18

A—Assemble a Support Group

Jesus was the original founder of support groups. He traveled all around Galilee and Nazareth gathering up people to follow Him, encouraging people to fellowship together, to help one another, and yes, to break bread together.

As we leave behind our dependence on food and grow to rely on God and on other important relationships, we will find strength in a unity of spirit with others. As Christians, we are never alone. We have Christ in us and we have a body of believers around us.

When our lives on this vast planet intersect, especially during times of intense personal change, the relationships we form in support group environments can be a most profound gift from God, lasting for a season or for a lifetime. Miraculous things can (and often do) happen when we sojourn together as a group to overcome any obstacle in life. This includes breaking negative habits and learning new patterns of behavior. It is in isolation that the devil can convince us of the lies that eating will make us feel better, that we deserve just one more bite, or that our circumstances are going to be impossible to overcome.

> There is a far deeper connection among those who sit together inside the same boat, frantically bailing water to stay alive, than with those who stand on the shore, no matter how encouraging they may be.

When we've used food as a false boundary and can finally look with complete honesty at our lives, we see that where our eating is concerned we have often acted in extremely irrational and self-destructive manners. Under the compulsion to overeat, over-diet, binge, purge, starve, or stuff, many of us have done things no sane person would think of doing.

It's good to know we're not alone in this realization.

> A strong wind is blowing across the church, and it is good. More and more churches are starting small group ministries. Some small groups meet for fellowship and support. Others meet to address specific life topics such as marriage, parenting, dating, addictions, or divorce recovery. Still others gather to study the Bible or to grow spiritually or even to engage in spiritual formation.
>
> One truth that has emerged from this small group movement is that there is no one right way to do small groups. Just as there are many mansions in God's house, so there are many different needs in God's body, the church, and today we are much more able to find a group somewhere that is designed to meet those needs.[1]

Throughout the years, some of my closest friendships have developed from support group settings. There is a far deeper connection among those who sit together inside the same boat, frantically bailing water to stay alive, than with those who stand on the shore, no matter how encouraging they may be.

There are two ways to assemble a support group. You can assemble in church or assemble in a small group environment.

Assemble in Church

The Christian life as described in Scripture is to be lived within the context of the family of God and not in isolation. Hebrews 10:25 is very specific when it teaches, "And let us not neglect our meeting together, as some people do, but encourage one another, especially now that the day of his return is drawing near."

The Bible teaches that it's important for believers to gather together to encourage one another, which gives every follower of Christ the job of being an encourager as well. This fellowship of giving and receiving is vital. It is also in attending church that we become equipped to be all God wants us to be, as Ephesians 4:11-16 so beautifully describes,

> Now these are the gifts Christ gave to the church: the apostles, the prophets, the evangelists, and the pastors and teachers. Their responsibility is to equip God's people to do his work and build up the church, the body of Christ. This will continue until we all come to such unity in our faith and knowledge of God's Son that we will be mature in the Lord, measuring up to the full and complete standard of Christ.
>
> Then we will no longer be immature like children. We won't be tossed and blown about by every wind of new teaching. We will not be influenced when people try to trick us with lies so clever they sound like the truth. Instead, we will speak the truth in love, growing in every way more and more like Christ, who is the head of his body, the church. He makes the whole body fit together perfectly. As each part does its own special work, it helps the other parts grow, so that the whole body is healthy and growing and full of love.

Fellowship is not just camaraderie. As Christians this is one of our responsibilities in life, coming together with believers on a regular basis so we can be joined together, becoming a holy temple for the Lord.

Assemble in a Small Group Environment

While assembling in a church environment is important, the assembly of people who are meeting collectively to conquer personal strongholds and gain strength is equally important. There may be other issues in your life contributing to the challenges you're having. Likely, they are problems that are being addressed in various small groups and issue-related support group environments around the country.

Six Steps to SANITY Support Groups

A day seldom goes by that I don't receive an email from someone inquiring if there is a SANITY Support Group meeting anywhere in their city. Although we are unable to track where groups are currently meeting, you can visit our website where readers communicate on the SANITY

Support blog. I'm also conducting online SANITY Support Groups myself throughout the year and that information is available as well by visiting my website SettingBoundariesBooks.com.

The first SANITY Support Groups launched in 2008. Groups began meeting in homes, churches, businesses, and community centers. Based on the first book in the Setting Boundaries series, *Setting Boundaries with Your Adult Children*, our first 12-week program met with great success all across the USA and throughout the world, in New Zealand, South Africa, Canada, Japan, England, and Germany. Literally thousands of parents and grandparents have found hope and healing from the crippling epidemic of enabling adult children. As word spread and groups were formed around the country, both live and online, it was soon clear the Six Steps to SANITY were applicable to far more issues than just learning how not to enable adult children who were lost.

Setting healthy boundaries isn't just a prodigal child issue.

My prayer has always been to offer SANITY Support to men and women addressing the myriad issues that swirl around the central core of unhealthy boundaries. To find out if a Six Step SANITY Support Group may be meeting in your city, or for guidelines how to begin your own SANITY Support Group, visit our website at SettingBoundariesBooks.com.

Assemble Support Today

In Hebrews 10:24-25 it is written, "Let us think of ways to motivate one another to acts of love and good works. And let us not neglect our meeting together, as some people do, but encourage one another, especially now that the day of his return is drawing near." In my Concordia Self-Study Bible, the heading above this passage reads *A Call to Persevere*. I can't think of a better way to describe the heart motivation of brothers and sisters in support group settings. Fellow sojourners ready and willing to persist in spite of difficulties, although not always able—and that's what support is all about—sharing the burden when someone is unable to carry it alone.

If you feel the need to communicate with other people in your same situation, ask God to open the door for you to get connected. God already knows the plans He has for you to be in fellowship with others. Ask Him to reveal that knowledge to you, praying for wisdom and discernment to walk boldly in God's purpose.

Maybe the hunger is not a physical one. Maybe your craving arises from an emotional need. Are you lonely? Would the food you think you want be a substitute for the human warmth and compassion you need? How can you get in touch with other people on a meaningful level so you won't suffer from loneliness?...If loneliness is behind your hunger, pick up the telephone before you take the first compulsive bite. Hug a family member or a friend. Join a club.

Are you angry? Are you afraid? Are you bored? Are you depressed? Are you low on self-esteem? Will extra food make the bad feelings go away for more than a few minutes? Are those few moments of relief worth the subsequent remorse? Talk about the anger and the fear...Most of us need all the help we can get. Find someone else who needs *your* help. Emotions—positive and negative—will pass. And they will come again. Let's learn to go with the flow and not try to medicate ourselves with food. Let your feelings come alive and vibrate. Give way to laughter and to tears. Open yourself to beauty and new experiences. Take life straight, without a sedative.[2]

Chapter 19

N — Nip Excuses in the Bud

What are the excuses that repeatedly come into play concerning your relationships with food? My go-to excuse was always that I deserved a little treat now and then, whether as a result of a stressful day or as a reason to celebrate. It didn't matter—either one worked. Or there was always the good ol' standby: "What's the point? I've already cheated; I might as well finish off the bag."

Whatever your excuses are, write them in your notebook now. If you can't think of any excuses off the top of your head ask God for a dose of truthful revelation. Or just wait until your next trip to the fridge and identify the thought that is prompting the urge to nibble.

By now you've noticed that I'm serious about encouraging the spiritual discipline of asking God to reveal His truth to us. This is a practice that didn't come naturally to me, and it's still something I *intentionally* do, but I'm certain the day will come when that won't be the case. I know this to be true for two reasons. First, I have faith. Second, the reason I've been making this an intentional practice is because God revealed to me that He wanted me to rely more on Him and less on myself, and the only way to do that is to consistently ask Him to reveal truth to my spirit.

I love what Oswald Chambers has to say about this:

> Christian experience must be applied to the facts of life as they are, not to our fancies. We can live beautifully inside our own particular religious compartment as long as God does not disturb us; but God has a most uncomfortable way of stirring up our nests and of bringing in facts that have to be faced.[1]

There's an excuse that often impacts our ability not only to find freedom from the bondage of weight obsession, dieting, and food challenges, but also from nurturing our most important relationship.

The Excuse That Diminishes Our Most Important Relationship

You may recall that I came to know the Lord late in life, at the age of 35. In my early walk as a new believer, I treasured Bible study and looked forward to it daily. When I first discovered the wisdom contained in the Word, I was hooked. Because my initial hunger for knowledge was so visceral, I assumed spiritual discipline must be something you automatically acquired through salvation. Both were new to me, transforming my life in ways I'd never imagined possible.

However, while my hunger and thirst to know God has never dissipated, I'm sorry to say there have been seasons when I let the busy things—challenging things—take over my life, robbing me of quiet devotional time and keeping me from making God's Word a priority. The excuse goes something like this: "God understands how busy I am. There's no way He expects me to read my Bible and take quiet time to be with Him every day."

Drs. Cloud and Townsend address this in *Boundaries*:

> When some people read the Bible, they see a book of rules, dos and don'ts. When others read it, they see a philosophy of life, principles for the wise. Still others see mythology, stories about the nature of human existence and the human dilemma.
>
> Certainly, the Bible contains rules, principles, and stories that explain what it is like to exist on this Earth. But to us, the Bible is a living book about relationship. Relationship of God to people, people to God, and people to each other. It is about the God who created this world, placed people in it, related to people, lost their relationship, and continues to heal that relationship. It is about God as creator: This is his creation. It is about God as a ruler: He ultimately controls his world and will govern it. And it is about God as redeemer: He finds, saves, and heals his loved ones who are lost and in bondage.[2]

We know setting boundaries is about guarding our hearts and healing the relationships in our lives. To do that, we need to learn new behaviors and new standards by which to live. We need to *Nip Excuses in the Bud* if they justify our destructive patterns and keep us from walking in right relationship priorities. The only way we are going to understand what is a right relationship priority is to spend time with the Author of priorities—God.

Something happens to us inside when we read and study the Word. The Lord quickens our heart and changes us. He brings us wisdom, discernment, and strength. It's not enough to just read Scripture once in a while, or see it on a wall hanging, or read it on a bracelet. Reading the Word daily is as life-giving as ingesting food and water. It's all about learning, growing, and changing according to God's Word and how He works on us and in us.

What we know today will change, including our feelings, thoughts, perspectives, and knowledge base. What will not change is the Word of God.

> God's way is perfect. All the LORD's promises prove true. He is a shield for all who look to him for protection (2 Samuel 22:31).

The Excuse That Calls God a Liar

There are so many different excuses for why we live in bondage to poor choices, challenging situations, and painful circumstances. Yet as different as the excuses are, many begin with the same two words. These are two words we need to ask God to help us remove from our vocabulary—two words that cut right to the heart of God, telling Him we do not believe His Word, and calling Him a liar: "I can't."

In her book *Seeing Yourself Through God's Eyes*, June Hunt speaks powerfully to those detrimental words:

> For thousands of years a club has been in existence offering memberships throughout the world. It's a popular club, a prolific club. It's the *"I Can't Club."*

Under the bylaws, club members are required to make "I can't" statements with conviction: "I can't help but hate him after what he's done to me." "I can't quit this sin." "I can't forgive again!" Such fervor makes it sound as if each "I can't" statement is an unchangeable, universal law.

If you're a member, your pledge echoes the club's premise: No one can win over sin. You believe its promise: defeat is normal. And you promote its purpose: to fill each mind with futility...

Do you feel bound to a specific sin? Does quitting the "I Can't Club" seem impossible? As a child of God, the word *can't* doesn't have to control your life. Upon your salvation, He gives you the Spirit of God so that you will have the strength of God. He deals a deathblow to the "I Can't Club." He makes it possible for you to overcome any sin.[3]

Whatever your "I can't" excuses may be, God is ready, willing and more than able to help you face them, including:

- I can't stop eating in the car...*yes, you can.*
- I can't stop drinking caffeine...*yes, you can.*
- I can't deprive my family of fast food...*yes, you can.*
- I can't spend time or money on counseling to deal with my issues...*yes, you can.*
- I can't bear to remember that part of my past...*yes, you can.*

...For you can do everything through Christ, who gives you strength (Philippians 4:13).

When Excuses Stop Working

You'll find over time as you tune yourself in to the Six Steps to SANITY that you'll soon be able to quickly identify an excuse...your own as well as others'. Once an excuse is identified for what it really is—a way to justify and perhaps even avoid the truth—we can then address the real issue at the heart of the matter, whatever that issue may be.

Pray for God to reveal to your heart the seeds of excuses when they begin to form. That way, you can eradicate them from your life before they bloom.

Chapter 20

I — Implement a Plan and Define Boundaries

Although we may not have been responsible for some of the things that happened to us in the past, we *are* responsible for our future, and our future depends on the choices we make today to take full responsibility for every aspect of who we are.

Hope lies in learning to depend on God and to make intentional choices that will change our lives and not just perpetuate the status quo. Implementing a plan and defining boundaries is all about taking action. We can talk all we want about finding sanity, but until we're willing to do the necessary work to change, we won't see much of a difference. We're often held in the grip of conflicting desires, wanting what the world offers at an extreme cost, yet needing what God can freely give. When we learn what to let go of and what to grasp, our lives can go from broken to joyous—just that fast.

In order to implement a plan it's a good idea to put that plan in writing first. It can be a short-and-sweet bullet point list or a multipage strategy, whatever works best for you.

But Allison, I'm not a writer, you say. *I'm really not very good at things like this…*

Is that an excuse I hear? If so, nip it in the bud!

This written exercise is about change and commitment. It's about living an intentional life. As you write, pray specifically for the Lord to reveal what you need to address that you've been avoiding. What really needs to be on your plan? Grab your journal and ask Him that question now. Write down the thoughts that immediately come to mind.

What is it that you really want to do? Stop eating after seven o'clock at night? Make better shopping lists in order to make fewer trips to the grocery store? Learn how to read food labels? Get your family involved in learning what it means to glorify God in our bodies?

Whatever it is, put it in writing.

A critical component in setting boundaries with food is developing the habit of really listening to our hunger *before* we eat something. If you're feeling convicted this is something you need to do, include it in your plan. We've also established that another critical component is better understanding our own negative behavior and destructive patterns. This may include learning to say no, being loving yet tough, and learning to say what we mean and mean what we say. Are any of these issues you think should be incorporated into your plan?

This is the time to start getting specific about the changes you're going to make. It's truly a landmark moment when we can calmly and rationally give voice to the needs we have, even if that voice begins on paper.

Considering the Consequences

An important part of writing a plan will be the work you do in exploring the natural consequences that may occur as you enforce necessary boundaries. The more prepared we are, the more likely we are to hold firm in our resolve. For example, I wish I had prepared myself more for the period of mourning I experienced in the months after my weight loss surgery—mourning for the food I missed. It may sound silly to some, but when we decide to give up the unnatural and unhealthy foods that do not honor our bodies and glorify God, we feel uncertainty, we feel the instability of the shaky ground

> We're often held in the grip of conflicting desires, wanting what the world offers at an extreme cost, yet needing what God can freely give. When we learn what to let go of and what to grasp, our lives can go from broken to joyous—just that fast.

beneath our feet as we walk on unfamiliar terrain, and we feel—sometimes quite deeply—the loss of this dependable companion that for so long met our unmet needs in destructive ways.

But there is high praise to our Holy God in this mourning—because through it all we are learning how to feel!

We *feel* the uncertainty.

We *feel* the instability of shaky ground.

We *feel* the loss of dependence on food.

And the most miraculous feeling of all—we *feel* God's increasing love for us and the joy of independence from the bondage of food and dieting!

Saying no to a negative habit so we can say yes to a positive goal is possible. We have survival instincts hardwired within us. We must leave behind our dependence on food and rely on a growing dependence on God. Setting healthy boundaries allows our true selves to emerge. Living an authentic life is something to be relished, and it's never too late to implement a plan and define boundaries—to make choices that will change our lives. Trust that God *can* help us to see the way we have been avoiding the truth. Trust that He will provide what we need, safely bringing us to a place where we can voice our needs in loving, honest, and authentic ways.

Getting Your Family Onboard

Last but by no means least, if you're the Nutritional Gatekeeper in your family and feel called to make changes (drastic or moderate) to the food you serve, it's important you speak privately first with your mate and then together as a couple with your children. This isn't cruel and unusual punishment you're handing down, and it's not a prison sentence. This is an opportunity for your family to grow healthier in mind and body.

You can visit my website to download free copies of various family food plans and togetherness plans that you can tailor to your family's specific needs.

Remember, honoring God with our bodies isn't an option. It's a mandate from God.

> Don't you realize that your body is the temple of the Holy
> Spirit, who lives in you and was given to you by God? You

do not belong to yourself, for God bought you with a high price. So you must honor God with your body (1 Corinthians 6:19-20).

Addressing Rebellious Opposition

If your kids refuse to eat healthy food, demand fast food, have tantrums, or demonstrate an increasingly rebellious spirit in response to the nutritional changes you've implemented, you'll need to address the issue. As Christian parents, our responsibilities to the spiritual as well as the physical health and welfare of our children will not always make us popular with them. However, popularity isn't the goal God calls us to as parents, is it? June Hunt says, "Having the peace of Christ inside you is entirely different from being a peace-at-any-price person."[1]

That especially holds true in families, where firm but loving boundaries between parents and children are needed.

> Saying no to a negative habit so we can say yes to a positive goal is possible. We have survival instincts hardwired within us. We must leave behind our dependence on food and rely on a growing dependence on God.

Perhaps this is one of the issues you've been avoiding by distracting yourself with food and dieting. If you're feeling overwhelmed at addressing your concerns I encourage you to apply the S in SANITY and stop, step back, and realize that God isn't going to give you more than you can handle. He already knows this is an issue in your life and He's been revealing truth to you for quite some time. The fact that you are reading these words right now is proof of that.

If there are boundary challenges in your family now there will be boundary challenges in your family as your children grow up. Unfortunately, these types of problems tend to grow as our children grow. This is seldom something they "grow out of."

Please visit your local Christian bookstore or preferred online shopping site to pick up a copy of *Setting Boundaries with Difficult People* or *Setting Boundaries with Your Adult Children* for additional help in making changes that are not only going to change the story of your life but the lives of those you care about as well.

The Food Plan

This will be a short section, because there is no specific food plan—not really. *Setting Boundaries with Food* isn't about following any specific food plan or regimented program. It's about listening to the hunger and learning how to stop using food as a false boundary to avoid addressing painful feelings or difficult situations.

However, I understand the need to follow some kind of plan, so I'm going to include one below. Feel free to copy this and stick it to your refrigerator with a magnet.

SANITY Plan - First Steps

1. Ask God every day to reveal new truth to you.

2. Continue your written *Food and Feelings Journal.*

3. Follow the Six Steps to SANITY daily.

4. Weigh yourself every day as a healthy habit, just as you would brush your teeth and comb your hair, and no matter what the number, don't beat yourself up about it.

5. Remove all garbage food from your house (i.e., processed, artificial, fried, unhealthy).

6. Go grocery shopping and buy fresh, whole, nutritious foods.

7. Read labels and learn the difference between nutritious food and empty-calorie food that is chemically processed or contains lots of fat and sugar.

8. Decide that for a time you'll give up eating at all-you-can-eat buffets or restaurants that serve fast food.

9. Eat a healthy breakfast, lunch, and dinner, and several healthy snacks throughout the day. Consume smaller portions.

10. Do not count calories, carbohydrates, grams, or points.

11. Do not deny yourself. Trick your brain with "not right now."

12. Learn the difference between physical and emotional hunger. Eat when you are physically hungry.

13. Decide what you want to do with the rest of your life—and start doing it.

SANITY Plan – Life Steps

1. Continue writing in your *Food and Feelings Journal*.

2. Follow the Six Steps to SANITY daily.

3. Weigh yourself every few days. Is the number staying the same, going down, or up? Be aware of your weight, and write it in your journal from time to time.

4. Grocery shop primarily on the edges of the store. Steer clear of center aisles, where the snack foods are located.

5. Stay away from high-fat, high-sugar, and processed foods.

6. Stay away from all-you-can-eat buffet restaurants.

7. Stay away from fast-food restaurants.

8. Eat a healthy breakfast, lunch, and dinner, and several healthy snacks throughout the day.

9. Listen to the hunger. Eat when you are physically hungry—not emotionally hungry.

10. Make a vow to stop the insanity and get off the starve-overeat-repeat treadmill. Go on a no-deprivation diet. Don't deny your food cravings, but first listen to where they are coming from.

Although I personally think it's important that we eventually break free from diet programs that encourage us to keep written food, calorie, and weight charts, I'm also aware that in our journey to set healthy boundaries with food it's going to be important for some of us to follow a more regimented nutritional program for a while in order to understand what it is our bodies really need. If you're such a person, I would encourage you to see if a First Place 4 Health support group is meeting in your community. This is a Bible-based weight loss plan that's been used successfully by over a half million people. It's not another diet program; it really is a way of life. Or you can start a SANITY Support Group based on this book. Visit our website for more information at SettingBoundariesBooks.com.

Chapter 21

T — Trust the Voice of the Spirit

The T step in SANITY was originally *Trust Your Instincts*, but when explaining the step in presentations or interviews, or teaching it in SANITY Support environments, I always referred to it as "listening to the still, small voice of God." Throughout the writing of this book, God impressed on my heart that if I'm challenging readers to say what they mean and mean what they say, why wasn't I?

Therefore, the T step in SANITY is now *Trust the Voice of the Spirit*.

Revelation Often Comes Slowly

When I first became a Christian and was struggling with the dilemma of moving in with my fiancé, I clearly recall my pastor telling me that he would pray for me to have Holy Spirit wisdom about the situation. So young in my faith at that time, I couldn't begin to wrap my brain around how that could actually manifest itself in reality. I didn't get it, even though I should have.

Over twenty years ago when I walked into that church in Orange, California, the Lord pulled the rug out from under me, forcing me to my knees in my time of desperation and brokenness. There is no doubt it was the Spirit of God at work, so profound was the experience—so cataclysmic was the change in my heart and life. Yet I had to agree with Oswald Chambers when he said, "The Spirit is the first power we practically experience but the last power we come to understand...a man receives the Holy Spirit, his problems are not altered, but he has a Refuge from which he can deal with them; before, he was out in the world being battered;

now the centre of his life is at rest and he can begin, bit by bit, to get things uncovered and rightly related."[1]

Therein lies the key—"bit by bit to get things uncovered and rightly related."

Trust Your Spiritual Intuition

The Bible teaches us in Proverbs 3:5-6: "Trust in the LORD with all your heart and lean not on your own understanding; in all your ways submit to him, and he will make your paths straight" (NIV).

How does God do that—"make our paths straight"? By giving us spiritual wisdom and discernment as we walk in relationship with Him, growing in obedience, understanding, and love for who He is and what He has done for us.

Stopping long enough to listen to God and to what our hunger is really saying can transform our lives.

It all begins with trust.

If we trust in the Lord with all our heart, we must also trust what He teaches us about the power of the Holy Spirit:

> And I will ask the Father, and he will give you another Advocate, who will never leave you. He is the Holy Spirit, who leads into all truth. The world cannot receive him, because it isn't looking for him and doesn't recognize him. But you know him, because he lives with you now and later will be in you (John 14:16-17).

Trust the Voice of the Spirit but don't expect the Voice of the Spirit to speak audibly to you. For the most part God speaks to us in two ways: prompting and teaching. Promptings take the form of inspirations or urges that show us what to do, with whom, and when. Teachings help us relate properly to specific situations, providing clarification and attitude adjustment. In short, teachings help us develop and refine our spiritual perspective, showing the way to stable happiness, and promptings contribute more toward enhancing spiritual intuition or insight.

Trust the Voice of the Spirit but don't expect the Voice of the Spirit to address all of your concerns. Instead, the Spirit will give you the power to transform your character to that of Christ and to glorify God always in all ways. More than anything else, trust that the Voice of the Spirit wants to produce in us the *fruit* of the Spirit: love, joy, peace, patience, kindness, goodness, faithfulness, gentleness, and self-control, transforming us not for individual exaltation, but for the good of the whole Body of Christ.

When I'm walking in God's will for my life, I can clearly feel His power within me, and this often manifests itself in very distinct impressions of how I should respond, behave, and think. It's as though my "intuition" is a divine power, guiding me to do what is right. That's because it *is* a divine power. It's the Voice of the Spirit, and this powerful inside track guidance is available to each and every one of us who believes.

Let me tell you, when you're walking in Holy Spirit wisdom you're going to know it! When we're able to listen and follow the inner voice of truth and wisdom and conquer the demons of habitual poor choice responses, it's a victory to be celebrated!

However, this kind of listening takes spiritual discipline. Trusting your spiritual intuition and not worldly lies, emotional uncertainly, or even the head knowledge you may have becomes more natural as we understand God's truth and hide it in our hearts. We need to have our roots firmly established in the soil of God's nurturing foundation. We need to know the standard God has established for us as His children, and the powerful truth contained in His Word, so that when the voice of the Holy Spirit speaks to us, we can hear it loud and clear and trust it implicitly.

We've Silenced the Voice

As Christians it's important to make decisions about life and relationships that are in keeping with God's truth and to pray, asking God to teach, prompt, and impress on us His wisdom, giving us discernment.

We ask, ask, and ask, yet when it comes to listening we are a bit more cautious. Oftentimes we *know* what is right, but we allow external influences (such as emotions, excuses, other people, or the fear of possible consequences) to control us.

Dozens of parents in pain who responded to my questionnaire for my book on setting boundaries with adult children berated themselves for not paying more attention to the prompting of their intuition. One mother had a particularly bad experience when it turned out her adult child had been dealing drugs from her home. "I was such a sap to believe him, and what makes me even angrier is that I had a feeling in my spirit that something wasn't right," she said. "I just didn't listen to it."

An Enemy of the Spirit

More years ago than I care to admit, I used to watch a popular TV program called *Rowan and Martin's Laugh-In.* One of the regular comedy skits involved Flip Wilson who was always popping up exclaiming, "The devil made me do it!"

As we know, the devil is a very real and very dangerous adversary, nothing to laugh at, and if we're not diligent about understanding what God's Word tells us about countering his plans to make our lives miserable, his deceitful voice can fill us with lies, fear, self-loathing, and an easy entrance to sin.

Always pray for discernment that the voice you are listening to is speaking truth that is aligned with God's Word. The voice of the true Spirit will never reveal anything to you that is not wedded to the words of the Bible.

Living by the Spirit's Power

Let's end this chapter by immersing ourselves in God's Word. The passage that follows is from Galatians 5:16-26.

> So I say, let the Holy Spirit guide your lives. Then you won't be doing what your sinful nature craves. The sinful nature wants to do evil, which is just the opposite of what the Spirit wants. And the Spirit gives us desires that are the opposite of what the sinful nature desires. These two forces are constantly fighting each other, so you are not free to carry out your good intentions. But when you are directed by the Spirit, you are not under obligation to the law of Moses.
>
> When you follow the desires of your sinful nature, the results are very clear: sexual immorality, impurity, lustful pleasures, idolatry, sorcery, hostility, quarreling, jealousy, outbursts of anger, selfish ambition, dissension, division, envy,

drunkenness, wild parties, and other sins like these. Let me tell you again, as I have before, that anyone living that sort of life will not inherit the Kingdom of God.

But the Holy Spirit produces this kind of fruit in our lives: love, joy, peace, patience, kindness, goodness, faithfulness, gentleness, and self-control. There is no law against these things!

Those who belong to Christ Jesus have nailed the passions and desires of their sinful nature to his cross and crucified them there. Since we are living by the Spirit, let us follow the Spirit's leading in every part of our lives. Let us not become conceited, or provoke one another, or be jealous of one another.

Chapter 22

Y — Yield Everything to God

It's often easy to see God in the exceptional things of life that make our spirits soar, or in the crisis situations that bring us to our knees. But it's much more difficult to see God each and every day in the places in the middle—in the ordinary living of life. This requires a spiritual discipline that's beyond our human nature to acquire, a habit that can only come when we *Yield Everything to God* and trust Him to be the Lord of our lives. Again, Oswald Chambers has it right.

> When we come to a crisis it is easy to get direction, but it is a different matter to live in such perfect oneness with God that in the ordinary occurrences of life we always do the right thing.[1]

At some point, every Christian will have to release his or her problems to God and learn to trust Him for whatever happens.

When the "letting go" part has been accomplished in our heart and the "letting God" part becomes a focus of our life, something amazing begins to happen. We feel free. We may not even realize how binding a prison our fears had been to us until those fears are gone.

> Come close to God, and God will come close to you (James 4:8).

True Growth Requires Letting Go

In addition to being an author, Leslie Vernick is a licensed clinical social worker and the director of Christ-Centered Counseling for Individuals and Families. Day after day, she experiences firsthand the devastating effects our past has on our present. Underlying virtually every issue is the mistake many of us make in hanging on tightly to the reins of our life or the lives of others. Leslie knows that true growth requires letting go. In her book *The Emotionally Destructive Relationship*, she writes,

> When we attempt to accomplish greater emotional and spiritual work, we usually think about the all things we need to *add* to our lives. We want to read and study the Bible, do meaningful ministry, gain greater emotional stability, better our interpersonal skills, or seek additional wisdom. All these endeavors can be helpful in our maturing process. But I have found in my own life as well as in my counseling practice that deeper and more lasting change usually comes about when we regularly practice letting go rather than doing more.
>
> Recently I was speaking with Richard, a client, who feared God's judgment when he died because he wasn't working harder to do more. As we talked I said, "Perhaps we've gotten the concept of final judgment wrong. What if, in the end, Jesus isn't going to tell us everything we've ever done wrong or failed to do? What if he's going to show us the person we could have become and the things we would have done if only we allowed him to heal and mature us?"[2]

True healing begins when we make the head-heart connection that we must "let go and let God" concerning all things, not only the painful situations that often occur in our lives. Leslie writes more about this in her book;

> Letting go in order to grow can be scary. It requires change, which demands a certain degree of faith and hope. That's why our picture of God must heal, at least a little, before we can embark on greater growth.
>
> The writer of Hebrews reminds us that we can only let go and run the race of life well when we keep our eyes on Jesus. Abiding and surrender…continue to be important as we practice the discipline of letting go.[3]

To "Yield Everything to God" does not mean we have given up. It is not a sign of defeat or weakness, but is, in fact, a sign of victory.

Chapter 23

How to Practice SANITY

It's important to keep any man-made program we may follow in the proper perspective, no matter how spiritually sound it may be. Finding SANITY isn't the end result, but a means to an end—with the end being a more intimate heart-relationship with Jesus Christ and a passionate desire to read His Word and understand His truth that will continue developing for life. There is a fundamental truth underscoring the deepest parts of our hearts. We were created for one basic purpose: to love and be loved by God.

Healthy boundaries do not develop in a vacuum, or in isolation. They develop as *we* develop—and we develop as we grow in the character of Christ, acknowledging God's love and sovereignty and depending on His sustaining grace, mercy, and forgiveness.

I'm often asked about my son, how he's doing.

Today, Chris is out of prison and remains drug-free. We are working to restore a relationship that has been ravaged by poor choices, addictions, incarceration, and estrangement. What does forgiveness really look like? How do we learn to trust again? How can families heal and build new memories after setting healthy (and sometimes very painful) boundaries?

One day at a time.

With God's help.

Oswald Chambers again:

> Take time. Remember we have all the time there is. The majority of us waste time and want to encroach on eternity. "Oh well, I will think about these things when I have time." The only

time you will have is the day after you are dead, and that will be eternity. An hour, or half an hour, of daily attention to and meditation on our own spiritual life is the secret of progress.[1]

The tangible result of finding SANITY is finding a new you and a new life.

Will you continue to operate "business as usual"? Will you keep allowing your hunger to control you? Will you continue to stuff down the pain with food and avoid the heart-issue at the heart of your issue? Or are you ready to take time to apply these Six Steps to SANITY and ask the Lord to help you make changes that will transform your life?

The choice is yours.

"Choose for yourselves this day whom you will serve..." (Joshua 24:15 NIV).

ALLISON'S TOP 10 SUGGESTIONS FOR SETTING HEALTHY BOUNDARIES WITH FOOD

1. Get a hard copy version of the Holy Bible (online versions are great, but not the same). Unless otherwise noted, I've used the New Living Translation (NLT) in this book. Ask God to reveal His truth to you as you study His Word daily.

2. Make journaling a part of your life. Writing even a sentence or two is better than writing nothing. Keep a notebook with your Bible.

3. If you don't have one, buy a bathroom scale and weigh yourself every few days. Don't be obsessed about this, but don't be in denial either.

4. Go on a search and destroy mission and get rid of all the unhealthy food in your home, including high-sugar, overly processed, and chemical-laden food.

5. Food labels are designed to give information about the nutritional content of the item. Learn how to examine a food label and interpret the information it provides.

6. If you are the Nutritional Gatekeeper for your family, discuss with them your plan to begin implementing better food and better nutrition into their daily regimen.

7. Get a hobby. Pursue your dream. Find what you love to do and do it. In short, get a life that exists beyond your weight, beyond food, beyond the challenging relationships you may have. Stop focusing on food and dieting.

8. Go through your closet and get rid of clothes that don't fit you. Anything that is too small or too big goes. Own and accept who you are now.

9. Listen to your hunger. What is it telling you? What emotions are you avoiding? What false boundary is food providing? Ask God to lift the veil from your eyes and reveal the steps you need to take to make healthy changes.

10. Practice the Six Steps to SANITY in conjunction with asking God to reveal His truth to you.

A Final Word from Allison

The closer we grow in our heart relationship with God, the more our hearts will grow with love for Him and what He is doing in our lives. When we understand that God says our bodies are the temples where He lives, it will become increasingly difficult to abuse that temple. When we cease using food to avoid feeling, depending more on God and less on food, our weight will eventually stabilize and maybe even begin to decrease. We'll have more energy, vitality, and strength of Spirit. Also, if we are the Nutritional Gatekeepers for our family's health, we'll be better able to supply them with what they really need to be the people God wants them to be.

As we pray for God to give us the one-day-at-a-time strength and wisdom to cope, over time our bodies and souls will heal. Oswald Chambers wisely wrote,

> Our bodies are to be entirely at God's disposal, and not God at our disposal. God does give Divine health, but not in order to show what a wonderful being a divinely healed person is. If God has healed us and keeps us in health, it is not that we might parade it, but that we might follow the life of God for His purposes.

Ultimately, that is what the Six Steps to SANITY can help us achieve on a daily basis—an understanding that as Christians our bodies do not belong to us and we need God's grace and power to get and stay healthy, so that "We might follow the life of God for His purposes."

You, too, can find SANITY, set healthy boundaries, and take back your life. Remember, God will always make a way where there seems to be no way. He is the author of our U-turns, new beginnings, and healthy boundaries!

God bless and keep you!

—*Allison*

Notes

Chapter 1 – Reorganizing Our Relationships

1. Oswald Chambers, *The Quotable Oswald Chambers*, ed. and comp. David McCasland (Grand Rapids, MI: Discovery House Publishers, 2008), 59.

2. Henry T. Blackaby and Claude V. King, *Experiencing God: How to Live the Full Adventure of Knowing and Doing the Will of God* (Nashville: Broadman & Holman Publishers, 1994), 31.

3. David Wardell and Jeffrey A. Leever, *Daily Disciples: Growing Every Day as a Follower of Christ* (Uhrichsville, OH: Promise Press, 2001), 30.

4. Blackaby and King, *Experiencing God*, 2.

5. Anne Katherine, *Anatomy of a Food Addiction: The Brain Chemistry of Overeating* (New York: Fireside/Parkside, 1991), 15.

6. June Hunt, *How to Rise Above Abuse: Victory for Victims of Five Types of Abuse* (Eugene, OR: Harvest House Publishers, 2010), 171.

7. Blackaby and King, *Experiencing God*, 37.

8. Ibid., 73-74.

Chapter 2 – Understanding Our Responsibilities

1. Henry Cloud and John Townsend, *Boundaries: When to Say Yes, When to Say No to Take Control of Your Life* (Grand Rapids, MI: Zondervan, 1992), 25.

2. Allison Bottke, *Setting Boundaries with Your Adult Children* (Eugene, OR: Harvest House Publishers, 2008), 33.

3. Tiz Huch, *No Limits No Boundaries: Praying Dynamic Change into Your Life, Family, & Finances* (New Kensington, PA: Whitaker House, 2009), 46.

4. June Hunt, *How to Rise Above Abuse*, 86.

5. Hope Lyda, *One-Minute Prayers for Women* (Eugene, OR: Harvest House Publishers, 2004), 42.

Chapter 3 – Defining Our Boundaries

1. Cloud and Townsend, *Boundaries*, 276.

2. Ibid., 25.

3. Hunt, *How to Rise Above Abuse*, 13.

4. Anne Katherine, *Boundaries: Where You End and I Begin* (Center City, MN: Hazelden Foundation, 1994), 131.

Chapter 4 – It's All About Balance

1. "Ann Curry's Aha! Moment: The Pursuit of Happiness," by Crystal G. Martin, *Oprah Magazine*, November 2011, 54.

2. Dr. Debra D. Peppers, *It's Your Turn Now* (Kirkwood, MO: Impact Christian Books, Inc., 2001), 85.

3. Ibid., 84.

4. Chambers, *The Quotable Oswald Chambers*, n.p.

5. Huch, *No Limits No Boundaries*, 45.

6. Duke Duvall, *How to Conquer Giants* (St. Louis, MO: Light of the World Publishers, 2001), 105-107.

Chapter 5 – Basic Biology and Destructive Dieting

1. Peter Jaret, "Fat? Who Cares! These 1,600 Words Could Change Your Life," *MORE Magazine*, October 2011, 166.

2. Kerry Patterson, Joseph Grenny, David Maxfield, Ron McMillan, and Al Switzler, *Change Anything: The New Science of Personal Success* (New York: Hachette Book Group, 2011), 153-154.

3. Roy F. Baumeister and John Tierney, *Willpower: Rediscovering the Greatest Human Strength* (New York: Penguin Group, 2011), 218-219.

4. Ibid., 214-215.

5. Katherine, *Anatomy of a Food Addiction*, 44-45.

6. Rachael F. Heller and Richard F. Heller, *The Stress Eating Cure, Lose Weight with the No-Willpower Solution to Stress-Hunger and Cravings* (New York: Rodale Books, 2010), 4.

7. Katherine, *Anatomy of a Food Addiction*, 64-65.

8. *Listen to the Hunger* (Center City, MN: Hazelden Foundation, 1987), 45.

Chapter 6 – Our Mighty Memories of Food

1. Katherine, *Anatomy of a Food Addiction*, 3.

Chapter 7 – God Is Love—Food Is Not

1. *Listen to the Hunger*, 4.

2. Geneen Roth, *When Food Is Love: Exploring the Relationship Between Eating and Intimacy* (New York: Penguin Books USA Inc., 1991), 123.

3. Huch, *No Limits No Boundaries*, 36.

4. Leslie Vernick, *The Truth Principle: A Life-Changing Model for Growth and Spiritual Renewal* (Colorado Springs: WaterBrook Press, 2000), 94.

5. Max Lucado, *Grace for the Moment* (Nashville: J. Countryman, 2000), 17.

6. June Hunt, *Seeing Yourself Through God's Eyes* (Eugene, OR: Harvest House Publishers, 2008), 9.

7. Blackaby and King, *Experiencing God,* n.p.

8. Vernick, *The Truth Principle*, 20.

Chapter 8 – Experiencing Emotions

1. Donna Carter, *10 Smart Things Women Can Do to Build a Better Life* (Eugene, OR: Harvest House Publishers, 2007), 29.

2. Doreen Virtue, *Losing Your Pounds of Pain: Breaking the Link Between Abuse, Stress, and Overeating* (Carlsbad, CA: Hay House, Inc., 1994), 37.

3. Roth, *When Food Is Love*, 123.

4. *Listen to the Hunger*, 41.

5. Jillian Michaels, *Unlimited: How to Build an Exceptional Life* (New York: Random House, Inc., 2011), 33.

6. *Listen to the Hunger*, 54.

7. Bernis Riley, quoted in Allison Bottke, *Setting Boundaries with Difficult People: Six Steps to SANITY for Challenging Relationships* (Eugene, OR: Harvest House Publishers, 2010), 65.

8. Harriet Lerner, *The Dance of Anger: A Woman's Guide to Changing the Patterns of Intimate Relationships* (New York: HarperCollins Perennial Currents, 2005), 1.

Chapter 9 – Listening to the Hunger

1. *Listen to the Hunger*, 55.

2. Peppers, *It's Your Turn Now*, 90.

3. *Listen to the Hunger*, 67.

Chapter 10 – The Conviction of Sin

1. Chambers, *The Quotable Oswald Chambers*, 180.

2. June Hunt, *Counseling Through Your Bible: Providing Biblical Hope and Practical Help for 50 Everyday Problems* (Eugene, OR: Harvest House Publishers, 2008), 317.

3. Ibid., 322.

4. Chambers, *The Quotable Oswald Chambers*, 58.

5. Cloud and Townsend, *Boundaries*, 62

6. Blackaby and King, *Experiencing God*, 283.

7. Chambers, *The Quotable Oswald Chambers*, 58.

8. Blackaby and King, *Experiencing God*, 288.

Chapter 11 – Food Sense and Sensibilities

1. Martha Beck, "Stay Cool," *Oprah Magazine*, November 2011, 60.

2. "Company Profile," McDonald's Corporation, accessed July 12, 2011, http://www.aboutmcdonalds.com/mcd/investors/company_profile.html

Chapter 12 – The Eating Experience

1. Degen Pener, "Meals My Mother Taught Me," *InStyle Magazine*, November 2011, 336.

Chapter 13 – Dreams and Goals

1. Jillian Michaels, *Unlimited: How to Build an Exceptional Life* (New York: Random House, Inc., 2011), 40.

2. *Listen to the Hunger*, 27-28.

3. Jennifer Strickland, *Girl Perfect: Confessions of a Former Runway Model* (Lake Mary, FL: Excel Books, 2008), 126-127.

Chapter 14 – Making the Choice to Change

1. David Hawkins, *Dealing with the CrazyMakers in Your Life: Setting Boundaries on Unhealthy Relationships* (Eugene, OR: Harvest House Publishers, 2007), 205.

2. Dr. Sidney B. Simon, *Getting Unstuck: Breaking Through the Barrier to Change* (New York: Warner Books, Inc., 1988), 5.

3. Simon, *Getting Unstuck*, 27.

4. Laura Schlessinger, *Bad Childhood, Good Life: How to Blossom and Thrive in Spite of an Unhappy Childhood* (New York: HarperCollins Publishers, 2006), 2.

5. Diane Keaton, *Then Again* (New York: Random House, 2011), 92-93.

Chapter 16 – The Power of SANITY

1. Chambers, *The Quotable Oswald Chambers*, 112.

2. Ibid., 115.

Chapter 17 – S—Stop Your Own Destructive Patterns

1. Carole Lewis, *Stop It! Quit Sabotaging Yourself—and Start Living* (Ventura, CA: Regal Books, 2005), 9.

2. Leslie Vernick, *The Emotionally Destructive Relationship: Seeing It, Stopping It, Surviving It* (Eugene, OR: Harvest House, 2007), 119-120.

Chapter 18 – A—Assemble a Support Group

1. Henry Cloud and John Townsend, *Making Small Groups Work* (Grand Rapids, MI: Zondervan, 2003), 13.

2. *Listen to the Hunger*, 68.

Chapter 19 – N—Nip Excuses in the Bud

1. Chambers, *The Quotable Oswald Chambers*, 92.

2. Cloud and Townsend, *Boundaries*, 228.

3. Hunt, *Seeing Yourself Through God's Eyes*, 61.

Chapter 20 – I—Implement a Plan and Define Boundaries

1. Hunt, *How to Rise Above Abuse*, 10.

Chapter 21 – T—Trust the Voice of the Spirit

1. Chambers, *The Quotable Oswald Chambers,* 120.

Chapter 22 – Y—Yield Everything to God

1. Chambers, *The Quotable Oswald Chambers,* 111.

2. Vernick, *The Emotionally Destructive Relationship,* 119-120.

3. Ibid.

Chapter 23 – How to Practice SANITY

1. Chambers, *The Quotable Oswald Chambers,* 297.

Allison Bottke is the author of the popular Setting Boundaries®
series, including *Setting Boundaries with Your Adult Children*,
and the general editor of the God Allows U-turns® series and the
God Answers Prayer series. She has written or edited more than
26 nonfiction and fiction books. Allison is a frequent guest on
national radio and TV programs and has been featured on *Focus
on the Family, The 700 Club, The Dr. Laura Show, Good Morning Texas, Decision Today,* and others. Visit her at AllisonBottke.
com or SettingBoundariesBooks.com.

Other books in Allison's
Setting Boundaries® series…

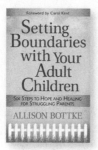

Setting Boundaries® with Your
Adult Children
*Six Steps to Hope and Healing
for Struggling Parents*

This important and compassionate book will
help parents and grandparents of the many adult
children who continue to make life painful for
their loved ones. Writing from firsthand experi-
ence, Allison identifies the lies that kept her, and ultimately her
son, in bondage—and how she overcame them. Additional real
life stories from other parents are woven through the text.

A tough-love book to help readers cope with dysfunctional adult
children, *Setting Boundaries with Your Adult Children* will empower
families by offering hope and healing through SANITY—a six–
step program to help parents regain control in their homes and in
their lives.

Foreword by Carol Kent (*When I Lay My Isaac Down*)

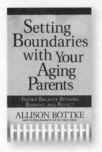

Setting Boundaries® with Your Aging Parents
Finding Balance Between Burnout and Respect

This important book from the author of *Setting Boundaries with Your Adult Children* will help adult children who long for a better relationship with their parents but feel trapped in a never-ending cycle of chaos, crisis, or drama. With keen insight and a passion to empower adult children, Allison charts a trustworthy road map through the often unfamiliar territory of setting boundaries with parents while maintaining personal balance and avoiding burnout. Through the use of professional advice, true stories, and scriptural truth, readers learn how to apply the "Six Steps to SANITY."

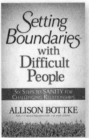

Setting Boundaries® with Difficult People
Six Steps to SANITY for Challenging Relationships

Continuing her Setting Boundaries series, Allison Bottke offers her distinctive "Six Steps to SANITY" to readers who must deal with difficult people.

Whether it's a spouse, in-law, boss, coworker, family member, neighbor, or friend, readers who have allowed others to overstep their boundaries will learn how these six steps can help them reset those boundaries and take back their life…for good.

Foreword by Karol Ladd.

And coming soon….

Setting Boundaries® with Teens:
Six Steps to Hope and Healing for Struggling Parents

To learn more about books by Allison Bottke or
to read sample chapters, log on to our website:
www.harvesthousepublishers.com